Walk Off the Weight

LUCY WYNDHAM-READ

WALK OFF THE WEIGHT

Fitness | Nutrition | Anti-Aging

21 days is
all it takes

Meyer & Meyer Sport

British Library Cataloguing in Publication Data
A catalogue record for this book is available from the British Library.

Walk Off the Weight
Maidenhead: Meyer & Meyer Sport (UK) Ltd., 2016
ISBN: 978-1-78255-077-8

© 2016 by Meyer & Meyer Sport (UK) Ltd.
Aachen, Auckland, Beirut, Cairo, Cape Town, Dubai, Hägendorf, Hong Kong,
Indianapolis, Manila, New Delhi, Singapore, Sydney, Tehran, Vienna
Member of the World Sport Publishers' Association (WSPA)
Manufacturing: Print Consult GmbH, Munich, Germany
ISBN: 978-1-78255-077-8
E-Mail: info@m-m-sports.com
www.m-m-sports.com

CONTENTS

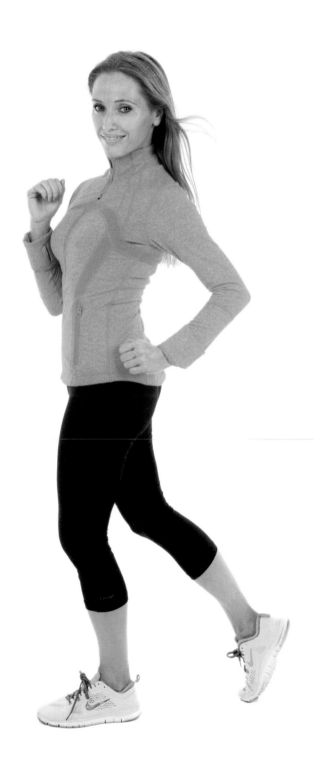

Part 1

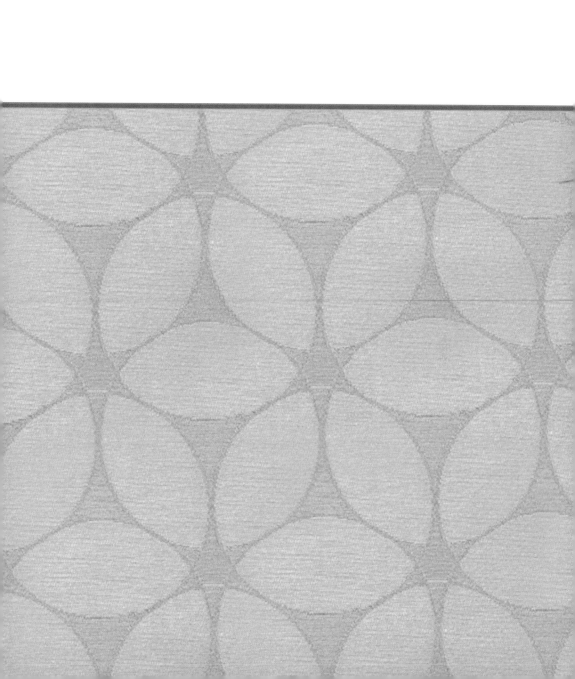

Part 1

INTRODUCTION: ABOUT LUCY

Lucy Wyndham-Read is a leading fitness and weight-loss expert with over 20 years of experience in the fitness industry.

She has helped hundreds of people reach their fitness and weight-loss goals. Lucy has her own highly successful YouTube fitness channel LWRFitness with over 1 million views and is an international fitness author and presenter.

Lucy creates her own workouts. From years of experience she has developed her own effective methods and created dynamic moves that engage several muscle groups all at once, resulting in workouts that are short and easy to follow. As a personal trainer, Lucy knows that most people haven't much spare time and get bored quickly when following the same routine. If they don't see results, they give up. So she has created quick, easy-to-follow and highly effective programmes. Once you start one of Lucy's workouts, you will be hooked on being healthy and fit for life.

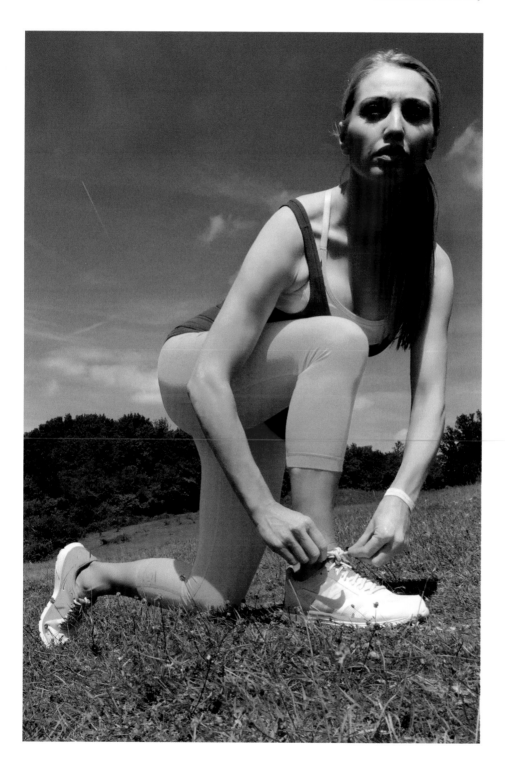

WHY WALKING WORKS

Walk yourself fitter, healthier
and younger.

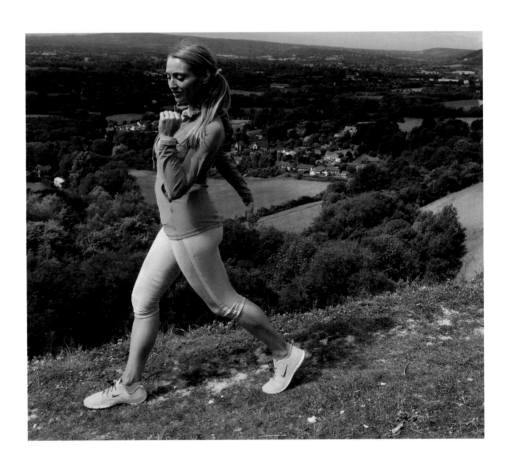

Walking is the most natural movement we do, and when we were children, it was the first exercise we ever undertook. Our bodies are designed to walk, and this low-impact activity suits every single fitness level, from a complete beginner who has never worn a pair of trainers to a budding athlete. The reason walking is the number-one exercise is that it engages all your major joints—ankle, knee, hip, elbows and shoulders—which means you are toning and recruiting big muscle groups—legs, butt, arms, abs, chest and back. When you walk, you burn lots of calories while at the same time sculpting and shaping your body. You can walk anywhere, it is free, and it is also very good for your soul. Even if don't have a garden or live by a main road, you are never far away from some pretty walks. Walking can also be fun to do with friends and family. Make it social, and you can spend good quality time with them and get fit at the same time. Going for a walk can be the new going out.

Walking is non-intimidating and so easy to follow, as it is simply putting one foot in front of the other. This is why it works, because it is our most natural exercise. It is suitable for everyone, and you can do it anywhere. You can even squeeze in a 15-minute walk on your lunch break. Walking is, hands down, a winner when it comes to your health, fitness, well-being, and body shape.

BENEFITS OF WALKING

Walking is the perfect exercise for every age.

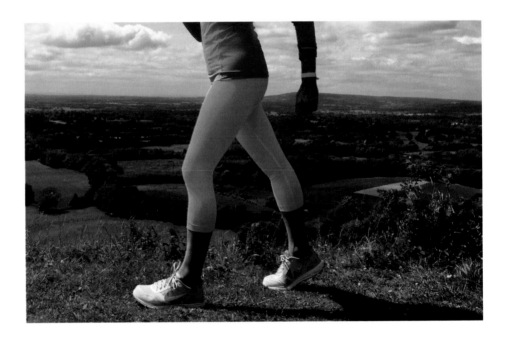

The list of benefits from walking is longer than you might expect. Your body reacts quickly to walking, and you *burn excess body fat, reduce inches all over, melt away muffin tops, sculpt and lift the butt, tone the thighs, and narrow the waist*. And you can wave goodbye to bingo wings. Even more important are the many other benefits to your **health, fitness, weight and aging** that walking provides.

So let's look at these in a little more detail, starting with **health**, which is the most important. Regular walking can help to prevent heart disease, type 2 diabetes, chronic illness, obesity, strokes, depression, and even some cancers. Read on to see how walking positively affects your health.

HEALTH

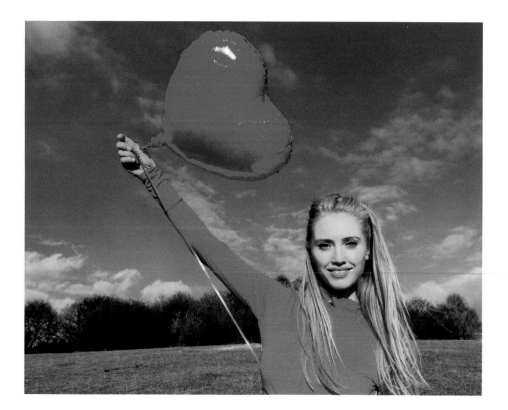

Strengthens the Heart

When we walk, we strengthen the most important muscle in our body—our heart. The stronger the heart becomes, the more effectively it works. The heart's job is to pump blood throughout the body. When a heart is weak (which can be due to lack of exercise), it becomes less effective at pumping blood. A good analogy I use is to imagine a foot pump that you are using to blow up an inflatable bed. If the pump is not very effective, you are going to have to pump it up and down lots of times for it to fill the bed. Yet if the pump is powerful and strong, just a few pumps will push in lots of air but with less effort. You want your heart to be a powerful pump so that with each pump it pushes blood through your system efficiently. The other benefit is that a strong blood flow keeps the arteries flushed and helps prevents them from narrowing, meaning you lower the risk of high blood pressure. Also the more effectively your heart pumps, the more oxygen it supplies to your body. So then you feel less out of breath and have more energy. This is why you should fall in love with walking, because your heart will love it, too.

Reduces Cholesterol

Walking is a great way to keep your cholesterol levels healthy, because walking at a brisk pace can help to reduce LDL (low-density lipoprotein). LDL is known as bad cholesterol that can cause a plaque lining in the arteries, and this can lead to heart attacks.

Prevents Osteoporosis

Stronger bones are essential for our frame and body support as we age. As we grow older, we can be susceptible to osteoporosis, which is a weakening within the bones that makes them more likely to fracture and break. Not only does walking tone and strengthen your muscles, but it also strengthens your bones, because every time your heel strikes the ground it produces a chemical process in your bones known as the *piezoelectric effect*. The piezoelectric effect helps to stimulate the cells that contribute to building stronger bones. This is why walking is a great way to keep your bones strong and healthy.

Prevents Obesity

Walking is a great way to keep your weight down and help prevent obesity, which also can lead to diabetes and other diseases. Simply put, when we walk, we use energy known as calories, and this is how we can stay in shape. Nowadays, obesity is a huge problem, and the reason is simple: People move less and eat more! If we sit all day—at the desk, in the car, shopping online—the body is not using energy, so it won't be burning calories. Instead we start storing calories and gaining weight, and this brings on a whole host of problems. But the good news is that by walking we can prevent all these health problems.

Lifts Depression

A great way to improve your mood and reduce stress levels is to go for a walk. Walking stimulates the production of the feel-good hormone known as *serotonin*. This is why when someone is suffering from depression, a doctor will often recommend walking, because it is the most natural way to help lift depression.

FITNESS

More Flexibility

Walking engages lots of muscle groups. With every stride we take (and this is true for each of my total-body moves), we use a full range of motion (ROM) through all our joints, which helps keep them healthy and flexible. Every time you engage a movement through a joint, you naturally increase lubrication knows as *synovial fluid*, which helps keep the joints smooth and mobile. Again, lack of exercise has the reverse effect, which is why joint problems can occur from inactivity.

Faster, Stronger, and More Stamina

Every time you work out, you increase the fibres in the muscles, making them stronger and increasing their endurance. Essentially your muscles can keep going for longer before they tire, and also they can carry more weight as they become stronger. The results of this are that you will feel fitter, and you will also find that you walk faster.

Better Balance

Walking, especially when you are walking outdoors over uneven surfaces, is a great way to work on improving your balance. You're naturally engaging what are known as the stabilising muscles, particularly around the lower legs, and this will lead to better balance. The total body moves I have created also have a huge impact on developing strong stability within your lower body, and overall you will notice a big improvement in your balance.

WEIGHT

Burns Calories

Walking can be a very easy way to manage your weight and even lose excess weight. The key is to walk at a very brisk pace, and with my walking workouts, we do just that. Completing my total-body moves has a great effect on weight loss. The reason is that we add short bursts of HIIT (high-intensity interval training). We use HIIT when we increase the speed of our walk, so the effort feels more challenging. These faster paces are between 20-40 seconds only, and then we bring the intensity back down. I will explain more later in the book, but what you need to know now is that this has an amazing effect on weight loss, because it produces an effect known as *EPOC (excess post-oxygen consumption)*. EPOC occurs when your body burns calories at a higher rate for hours after you have finished exercising. This can burn an extra 35 calories an hour and can stay at an elevated rate for up to 10 hours, so you can see why I get excited about this and why weight loss then becomes easy. That is going to be an extra 350 calories you burn even after exercising. This also applies to my total-body moves, as it tones so many muscles at once, and the more toned the muscles are, the more calories you burn.

AGING

Turns Back the Clock

Believe it or not, walking can turn back the clock. Exercising helps promote the hormone that is responsible for fighting aging—the *human growth hormone (HGH)*. In our late 20s, this hormone naturally starts to decline, resulting in the loss of plumpness and radiance in our skin. So as we age, our skin texture and appearance start to change. Basically, this hormone starts to retire at the end of your 20s! People pay fortunes to have injections which contain HGH just so they can improve the look of their skin, but the good news is that you can actually re-employ this hormone, and we do this simply by exercise. Exercise stimulates the production of HGH. Your body will then be producing this hormone back into your system, especially when you are exercising regularly. The result is that you boost your collagen levels, plumping up your skin, reducing fine lines and giving you back the radiance in your skin, whatever your age.

WHAT YOU WILL GET FROM WALKING

- Toned thighs
- Slimmer waist
- Lifted butt
- Increased calorie burn
- Stronger bones
- Better mood
- More energy
- Slimmer arms
- Reduced cellulite
- Less tummy fat
- Melted away muffin tips
- Banished bingo wings
- Plus all the other amazing benefits mentioned already.

This is why walking is about to become your number-one exercise!

1

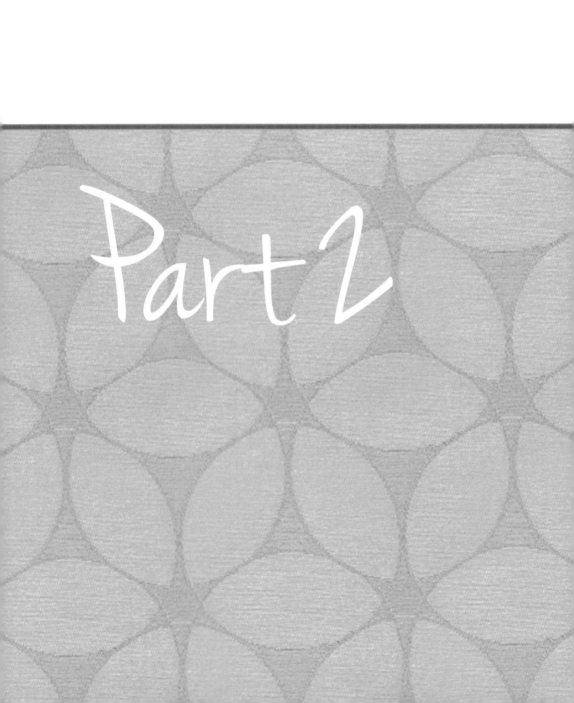

Part 2

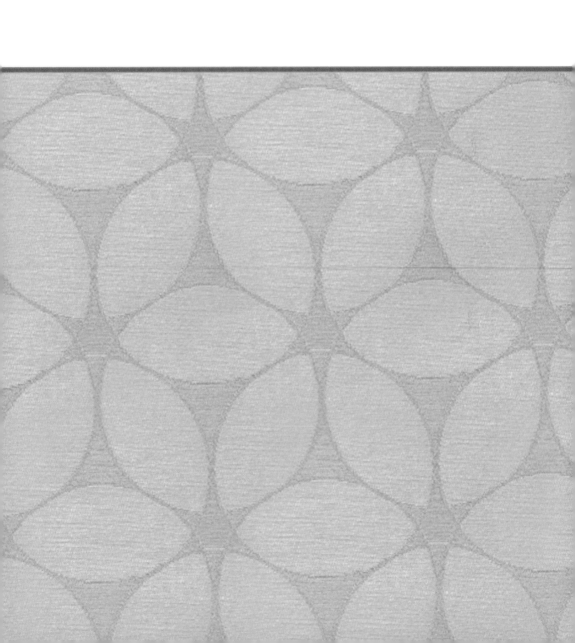

Part 2

WHAT YOU NEED

You will be following this plan for the next 21 days, and there are a few things that you will need.

WHAT YOU NEED TO WEAR:

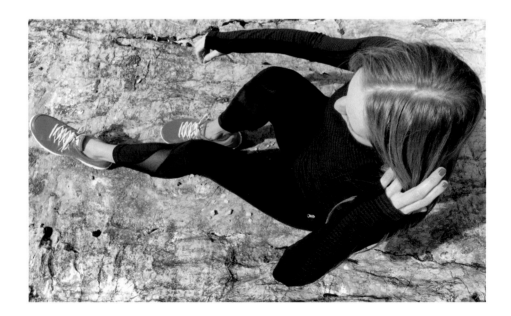

Trainers. A good pair of trainers is a must! These don't need to be expensive, but they do need to feel comfortable and have a good flexible sole. A good way to test the sole is to bend the trainer so that the toe section reaches close to the middle of the shoe. By being this flexible it means it gives you the range of movement you need to walk at a good pace, without the shoe being too structured around the foot.

Also, these trainers will be fine to use for the total-body moves that we will be doing throughout the week.

Sports bra. Even though this 21-day walking plan is all low impact, it is still very important to wear a well-fitting sports bra, because this helps support the bust as well as the muscles and ligaments around the bust area. Our bust can move in an up-and-down and side-to-side motion over a distance of up to 8 centimetres (3 in.) if we have no support, so this is why it is important to invest in a good sports bra—to secure the bust firmly in place while exercising. Also, it is much more comfortable.

As for the rest of your fitness gear, you don't need to go and spend lots of money on a whole workout wardrobe, as you can easily exercise in comfortable leggings, tracksuit bottoms or shorts and t-shirts. Layers are best. As you warm up, you can then peel them off to adjust to your body temperature. What is a must, though, is to select your brightest colours for when you are heading outdoors for a walk, because it is so important to always make sure you are highly visible. Additionally, in the summer you can always wear a hat, and look after your eyes by wearing sunglasses.

GADGET KIT LIST

This, again, is a very short list, but my few suggestions are definitely worth investing in, as these will have such a big impact on your results and ongoing healthy lifestyle.

Pedometer. These clever little devices keep track of how many steps you take and are a great way to encourage you to be more active throughout the day. Within the book I also give you certain step-count challenges. Doing a set amount in one day can have a whole host of positive benefits to your health and weight. So even after you have finished my

21-day plan, this will be a great tool you can use to help in easily maintaining what you have achieved. These are not expensive, and you can easily pick one up online or at any good sports shop. They can be less than the price of a cup of coffee! Also, nowadays, there is so much wearable technology with funky-looking bracelets and watches that not only tell you the time but also clock each step, and they even transfer the data collected to your phone! Also, there are lots of free apps you can download to your phone which monitor your daily step count. So a pedometer is definitely a must.

Spiralizer. I go on and on about these all the time and in most of my books. The reason is that it can so simply turn your vegetables into amazing dishes. The best example is courgettes. Courgettes can be spiralized so that, as if by magic, they turn into long spiral bands that can be cooked just like pasta (and taste just like pasta) but without the calories. There are lots of these online, and they are not expensive and definitely worth having in your kitchen if you want to enjoy eating easy-to-prepare healthy meals.

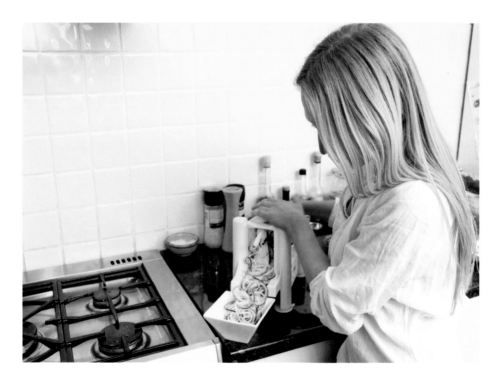

Water bottle. Okay, this is not a must, as let's be honest water comes in a bottle anyway, but if you want a little extra motivation to help ensure that you are drinking enough water daily, then spending a little money on one, say in your favourite colour, is a good idea. There are also some great ones that have filters.

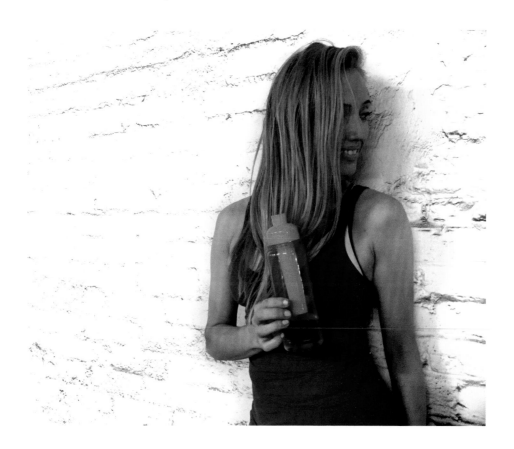

Any of these three items would be a great way to invest in your Fit Kit, and they prove how cheap and inexpensive being fit can be. There is no need for expensive bits of equipment, misleading dietary supplements, fad fitness products or gym memberships. So save your money and start enjoying getting fit the healthy way.

HOW THE PLAN WORKS

A plan I have always stuck by, and it's what makes my workouts effective, is the KIS method:

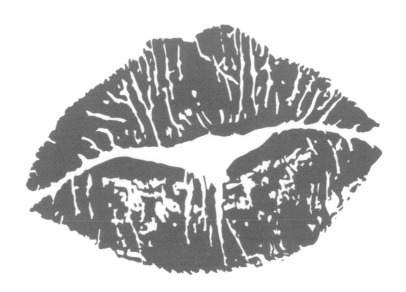

Keep. It. Simple.

By keeping it simple, you have 100 per cent confidence and clarity in what you are doing. All you need do is simply proceed with the plan day by day and follow the instructions shown. Each day for three weeks you will have a different set exercise which will either be a walking workout or a total-body toning move. The full description of each of these will be in detail at the beginning of each new week.

Then for your anti-aging, healthy-eating plan, you just aim to stick to the meals and snacks I recommend on that day.

So you can see it is that simple.

Simply follow the instructions for each day.

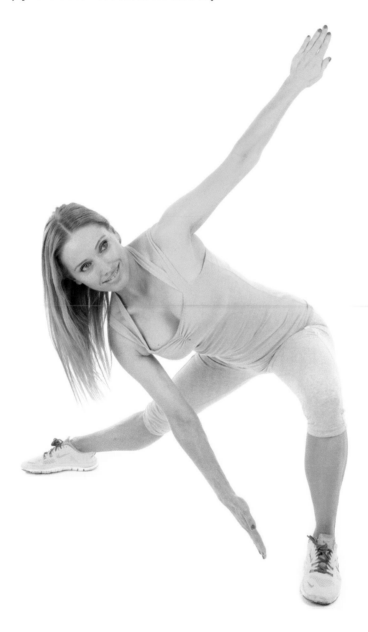

HOW THE WALKING ROUTINES WORK

Each week I set you a new walking workout, and we will focus on adding a sculpting move to that walk. But firstly, before we look at that, let's establish how to put some power into that walk and how to do it with good form.

It's all about the pace, as walking along at a leisurely stroll is not going to gain us the results we want; we are going to have to take it to a brisk pace. A good way to monitor your pace is with the walk fit gauge.

Walk Fit Gauge

Level 1 = an average pace at which you would walk around a supermarket.

Level 2 = a slightly faster pace than level 1, but you would still be able to hold a full conversation on your mobile phone whilst walking.

Level 3 = a brisk pace, and you would not be able to hold a full conversation but rather only answer with a yes or no. You would feel slightly out of breath. You have now hit the jackpot, because this is the optimal walking speed you need to get all the health, fitness and weight-loss results.

Level 4 = walking so fast you are locking out all your joints and look similar to the road-race walkers. You feel so out of breath you can't speak! Well this is too much, and you need to reduce that pace back down to level 3.

DIFFERENT STYLES OF WALKING

Each week I will set you a new walking workout challenge and this will consist of short intervals in which we vary your walking style.

HOW TO DO THE DIFFERENT STYLES OF WALKS:

Brisk Walk:

This is a good fat burner.

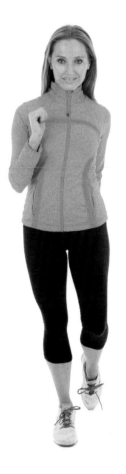

2

Simply focus on walking with a good brisk pace in every stride.

Ab Toning Stride:

This is great for toning your abs.

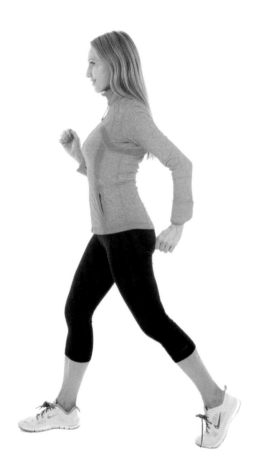

Walk with a slightly shorter stride and focus on keeping your tummy muscles pulled in. Ensure you keep your shoulders stacked over your hips.

Faster Walk:

This is great for increasing your calorie burn.

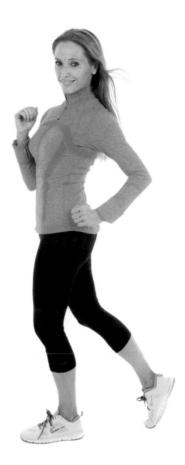

Take a slightly shorter stride and focus on pumping with your arms. The faster you pump your arms, the faster you walk.

Deeper Stride:

This is great for toning and sculpting deep into your hips, bottom, and thighs.

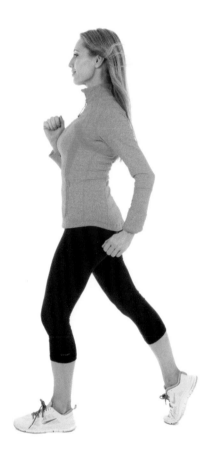

Focus on taking a slightly deep stride, so you really extend your leg out behind you. You will instantly feel this lifting and toning your butt. Ensure that you still maintain good upper body posture.

Arms Crossed Stride:

This tones and shapes your abs and butt.

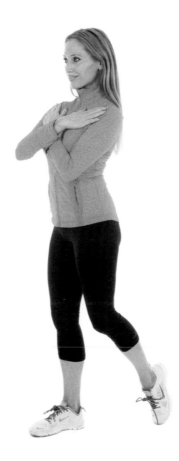

Walk at a good, brisk pace and simply have your arms crossed and resting on your chest. This means that all the power used to walk is coming from your legs, butt, and abs. Keep focussing on taking your normal walking stride and keep your upper body straight.

INTENSITY

Above, I have mentioned my Walk Fit Gauge. This guide helps you understand how you can always ensure that you're walking at the right speed to get maximum results.

But for your walking workouts, I want to focus on doing short bursts in which we really push up the intensity of the workout. It is the intensity that really helps melt away body fat and get us great results.

Gauging exercise intensity can be difficult, expensive, and time-consuming, yet all you need to do is learn about and adapt one of the best-kept secrets of the fitness world: THE RATE OF PRECEIVED EXERTION SCALE. This RPE scale simply allows you to monitor the level of intensity you are training at so that you can ensure that you are working out at the correct intensity for your walking workouts.

I suggest you familiarize yourself with this scale because we will refer to these levels throughout the book, and each individual workout lists the RPE level you should be training at.

RATE OF PRECEIVED EXERTION SCALE

1   Nothing at all (sitting on the sofa)

2   Very, very light

3   Very light (gentle exercises)

4   Moderate

5   Somewhat hard (feeling a little out of breath)

6   Hard (unable to hold a conversation)

7   Very hard

8   Very, very hard

9   Near exhaustion

10   Maximum

Note: We never need to enter level 9 or above, and exercising at those levels is not recommended.

So now that we have established the speed, let's look at how to walk with good form and posture. (You can also visit my YouTube Channel and watch the video called "How to Power Walk.")

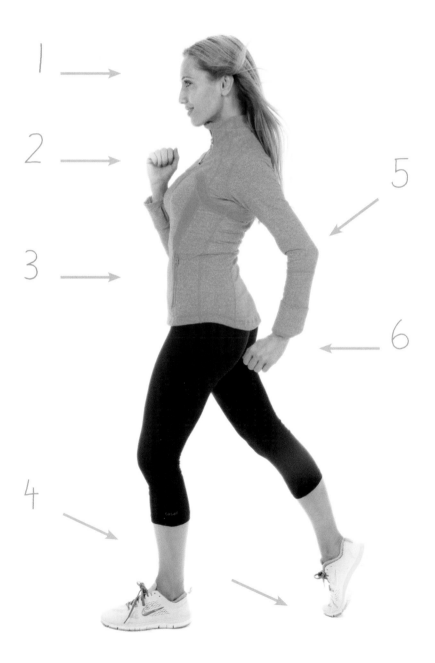

1. You should keep your chin parallel to the floor, and you should be focusing your eyes 5 to 6 metres (15 to 20 ft.) in front of you.

2. Maintain good upright body posture

3. Gently pull in your tummy muscles.

4. Always land on your heel, and then roll through your foot, pushing off from your toes.

5. Avoid swinging your elbows higher than your breastbone, and keep them in a relaxed bent L shape.

6. Focus on keeping your pelvis under your torso.

7. And lastly, remember, to turn it into a power walk you need to be walking at level 3.

HOW THE TOTAL-BODY TONER MOVES WORK

No need to spend a long time toning; instead do one of my toning moves that targets all major muscles at once!

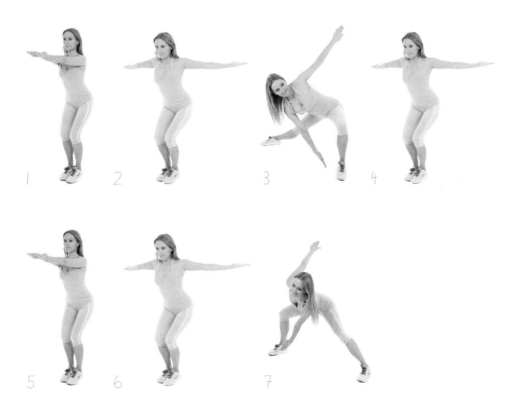

Each week I give you a new move called a *total-body toner*. It works all major muscles groups—bottom, thighs, abs, chest and arms—in three directions—forwards, sideways and laterally. This is why I also refer to it as a multi-gym move!

The great thing with these moves is that they save you heaps of time, because you are toning all over. Again, the workouts are super simple to follow.

2

Keep. It. Simple.

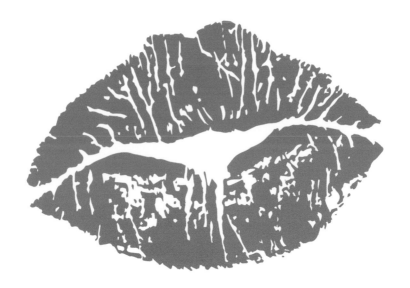

At the beginning of the week, I give you a goal to perform a set number of that specific move, and each day we increase the amount of times you perform the exercise. Throughout the three weeks, the goals will get progressively harder, but that is because you will be getting progressively fitter.

Fact: When we do an exercise that engages multiple muscles groups, we turn the body into a fat-burning machine instead of a fat-storing machine.

ABOUT THE ANTI-AGING EATING PLAN

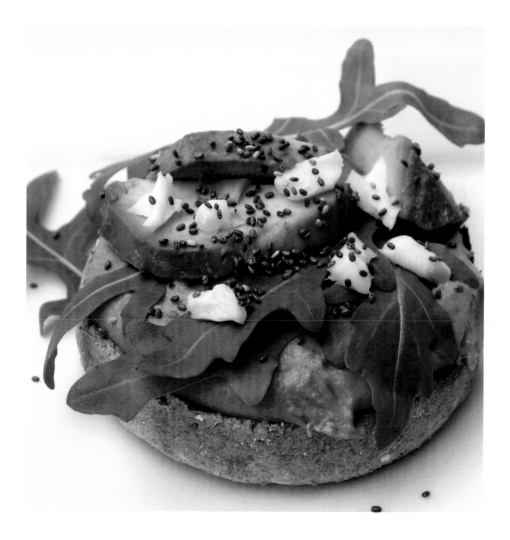

One of the best ways to look as if you have just arrived back from a week's visit to a health spa is to be smarter with your fork. By this I mean that if we eat a diet rich in vitamins, antioxidants and minerals, we will be glowing with radiance and health from the inside

2

out. As well as giving us plenty of energy and preventing us from feeling bloated, our food is meant to be enjoyed, and I hope that the 21-day eating plan will show you how easy and enjoyable it is to eat *clean*—in other words, no processed food.

Some of the benefits of following this 21-day plan are the following:

* **Smoothing out fine lines.** We do this by eating antioxidants that are fat soluble and sit in the upper layer of your skin; these antioxidants help to plump up the skin and to protect and nourish your cells.

* **Hydrating your skin.** We hydrate by eating foods that help your body hold on to moisture for vital healthy glowing skin.

* **Reducing breakouts and spots.** These are often brought on due to too much oil released from the sebaceous glands. With this eating plan, we focus on foods that are high in minerals to help keep the glands in check.

HOW TO WARM UP, STRETCH AND COOL DOWN

Before your walks or total-body toning moves, it is always important to warm up, and after your workouts, it is important to stretch and cool down. Warming up will help you perform the exercises safely and help internally warm up your muscles and joints. The benefits of a warm-up are that it helps prevent injuries and helps your muscles become more pliable, meaning you feel more mobile and are able to perform the exercises with a bigger range of movement, which is very important in order to get the best out of each exercise.

You should always spend a couple of minutes warming up. If you are doing the total-body move, then your warm-up could be as simple as marching in place or walking up and down the stairs. Then for your walking workouts, just spend a minute or so walking at a slower pace to gently increase your core body temperature. The important thing is to make sure you feel warm before you start. My advice is to perform all the stretches that I recommend here at the end of the warm-up. And at the end of your workout, just march it out for a minute or so to slowly bring your heart rate back to its pre-exercise state, and then perform the stretches again as part of the cool-down. This will help prevent any injuries and will also help realign the muscles after training.

Thigh Stretch

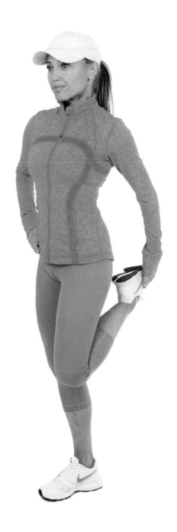

Standing with good posture, bend one leg behind you and gently hold the foot of the bent leg. Push your hips forwards to feel the stretch in the front of your thigh. Keep the supporting knee slightly bent. Hold the stretch for 10 seconds on each leg.

Calf Stretch

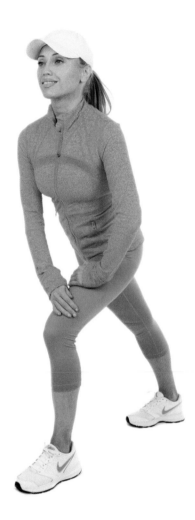

Step back with one leg, keeping the heel down and both feet pointing forwards. Rest your hands on the bent leg. Hold the stretch for 10 seconds on each leg.

2

Hamstring Stretch

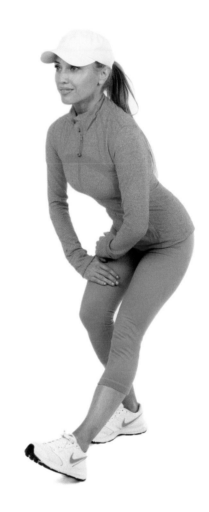

Standing straight, bend one leg and extend the other out straight in front of you with heel on the floor and toes pointing up. Place both hands on bent leg and stick your bottom out to feel the stretch along the back of the straight leg. Hold the stretch for 20 seconds on each leg.

Chest Stretch

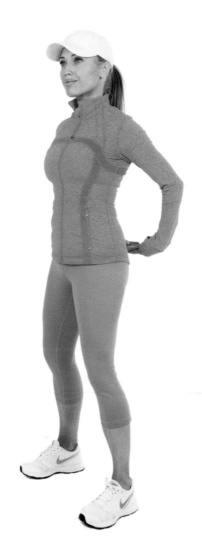

Standing with good posture, take your arms behind you. Clasp your hands and lift your shoulders up and back to feel the chest stretch. Hold the stretch for 10 seconds.

Back Stretch

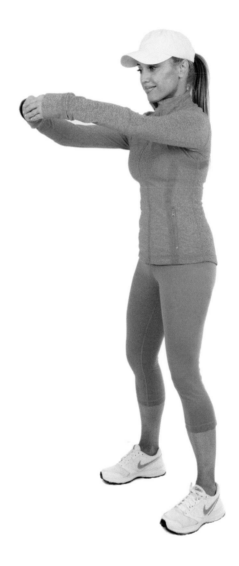

Stand with good posture, knees soft and tummy pulled in. Take your arms in front of you and clasp the hands together. Imagine you are hugging a big beach ball to feel the stretch in your back. Hold the stretch for 10 seconds.

Triceps Stretch

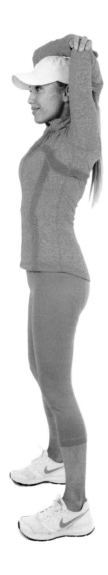

Stand with a strong, firm, straight back, knees slightly bent and tummy pulled in. Lift one arm up and bend it behind your head, keeping your upper arm close to your ear while aiming to get your hand between your shoulder blades. Hold the stretch for 10 seconds.

2

HEALTH AND SAFETY

It is vital that you always put your health, safety and wellbeing first, so always apply these following rules:

Never train if you are feeling unwell.

Never train if you have an injury.

Avoid always using the same route at the same time on the same day.

When training outdoors, always take a phone with you, and let someone know where and when you are going.

Always wear highly visible clothing when you are walking.

Always wear sunscreen and a hat if you are training in the sun.

Always keep yourself fully hydrated.

Always stick to well-lit and unsecluded pathways.

Always carry a small snack and bottle of water with you.

Always wear the right training gear.

Always warm up, stretch and cool down after every workout.

WALK FIT TEST

As you will be increasing your fitness, it will be nice to see how well you have done. So before you start the 21-day plan, I suggest that you find a route that is exactly **0.5 miles**. Walk this route as fast as you can and make a note of the time it takes you to complete it. Also take a note of how you felt after it—for example: exhausted, hot or easy. Then redo this test in 21 days' time. You will see that you now complete the route faster, and you will see how much you have increased your fitness.

Date (prior to the plan)	Route 0.5 miles
Time taken:	How you felt:
Date (after 21 days of the plan)	Route 0.5 miles
Time taken:	How you felt:

MEASURE IT AND SNAP IT

Seeing progress is one of the best motivators. Each week you will be reducing excess body fat and dropping the inches, so you may want to measure yourself to see just how many inches are coming off. Another way to view progress is to take a selfie at home. Stand in front of the mirror in your underwear or fitness gear and snap away. Also do a couple from the side. Each week you will see your body tone up and tighten in these pictures.

To take your measurements, I suggest you measure your waist by placing tape measure around the narrowest part of your waist.

Then measure your bottom at the widest part.

Also measure your thigh and arm. Choose the same side, either the left or right, to measure each time. For your thigh, measure a quarter of the way down, and then do the same for the arm.

Week 1	Measurements
Waist	
Bottom	
Thigh	
Arm	

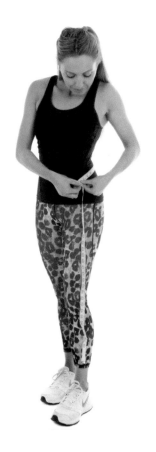

What to Expect by Day 7

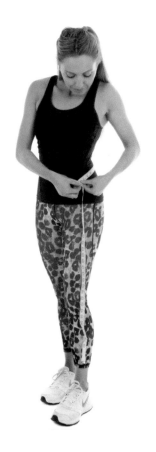 You should notice that the inches are starting to come off, most probably around your waist and hips.

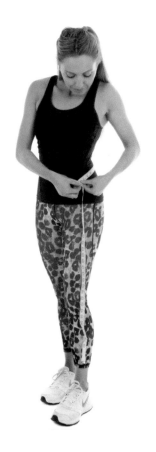 You will have more energy.

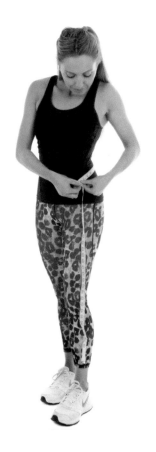 You will find that you are sleeping better.

What to Expect by Day 14

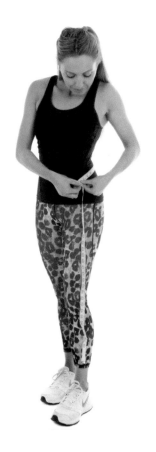 You will probably find that you have now gone down a dress size.

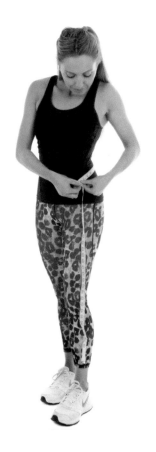 You will be walking faster and feeling so much fitter.

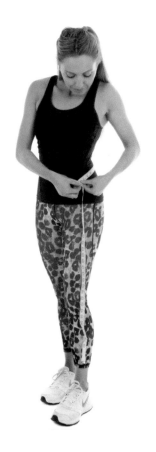 You will notice that your skin looks firmer and is glowing with radiance.

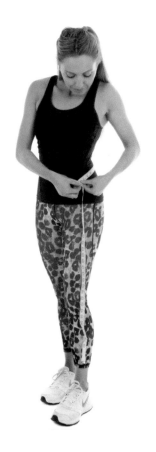 You will notice you feel stronger when you are doing your total-body move.

2

What to Expect by Day 21

- You should now be getting compliments from everyone, because you will look so good.
- You will have dropped a dress size, or maybe even two.
- You will have lifted and sculpted your body.
- You will have reduced any cellulite, if you had any.
- You will find when you redo your Walk Fit test that you complete it so much faster and feel so much fitter for it.
- You will simply feel amazing and be so pleased you did this for the last 21 days.

COMMITMENT

Before we start there is just one thing you need to say to yourself:

'I AM GOING TO DO THIS'

It is the consistency that will get you results. You need to apply some **discipline** and **determination** and just say: 'For the following seven days I am going to stick to this.' (Even though it is 21 days in all, let's always just break it down to 7 days.)

Part 3

Part 3

WEEK 1

MOTTO FOR WEEK 1:

Start like you mean it.

16-MINUTE INCH-LOSS WALKING WORKOUT

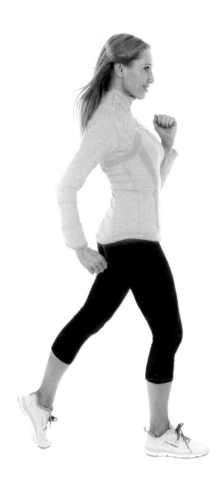

16-Minute Inch-Loss Walk

Time	Walk style (see page 29)	Intensity (see page 34)
2 minutes	Brisk Walk	5
1 minute	Ab Toning Stride	6.5
1 minute	Deeper Stride	6
Repeat this sequence 4 times.		

3

TOTAL-BODY TONER FOR WEEK:
REACH FOR THE STARS LUNGE

This move is called the **Reach for the Stars Lunge**. It was named by @lottierainbow on Instagram.

The **Reach for the Stars Lunge** tones your thighs, bottom, abs and arms, meaning you are going to be toning all over while also engaging so many muscles groups in this one exercise that you will be supercharging your metabolic rate.

How to do it:

- Start by standing in a split stance with the heel of your rear leg slightly raised off the floor and extending both your arms directly above your head with your palms pressed together.
- Pulling in your tummy muscles, slowly start to bend through your knees as if you are aiming for the back knee to reach the ground. At the same time, bend your arms and aim for your hands to reach in-between your shoulder blades. Hold this position for a second before slowly pushing back up to your starting position.

Throughout week 1 you will see the amount of repetitions I recommend you do on the set days, and each time I will be increasing the repetitions slightly, as your body becomes fitter each time you perform this move. (You can see the full instruction video "How to the reach for the Stars Lunge" on my YouTube Channel.)

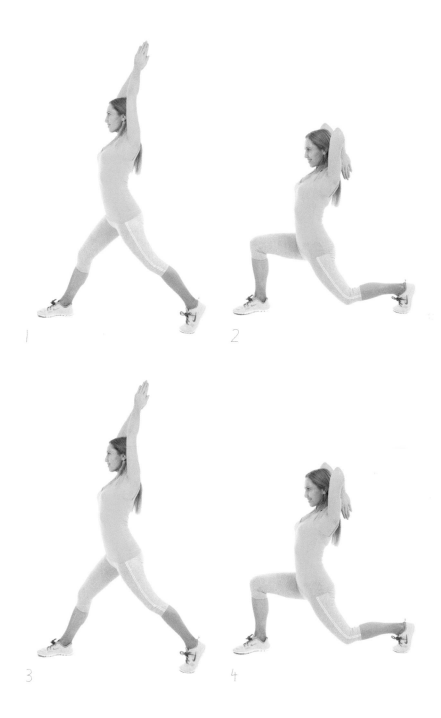

1

2

3

4

DAY 1

EXERCISE

16-Minute Inch-Loss Walk (see page 59)

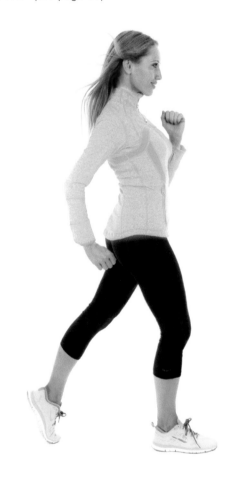

MENU

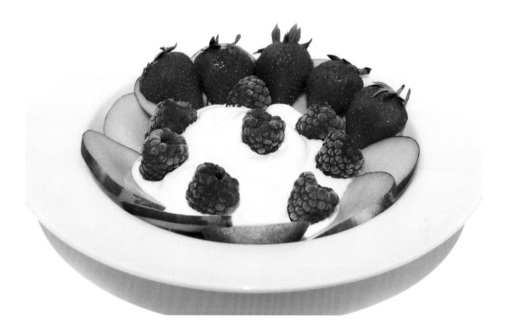

Breakfast: Small low-fat yoghurt with sliced strawberries, nectarine and raspberries

Snack: Celery sticks and added low-fat cream cheese topped with a sprinkling of poppy seeds

Lunch: Wholemeal pita filled with tuna (spring water), rocket and chopped red peppers; 1 banana

Snack: Cucumber sticks with small amount of hummus

Dinner: Grilled lean steak served with steamed spinach and sweet corn

DAY 2

EXERCISE

Total-body move: Reach for the Stars Lunge. Complete 12 reps on each leg.

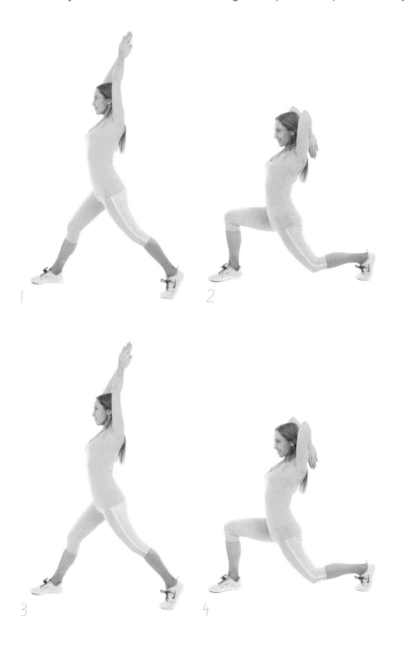

MENU

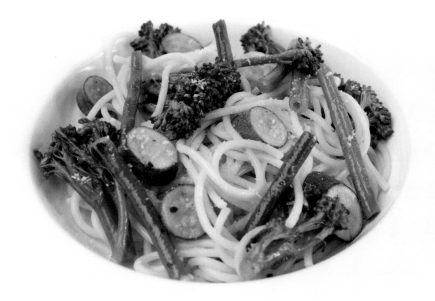

Breakfast: Small bowl of whole-grain cereal with semi-skimmed milk and chopped banana

Snack: Sliced strawberries with cottage cheese

Lunch: Open wholemeal chicken breast sandwich with avocado, tomato and lettuce salad; low-fat yoghurt

Snack: Small handful of cashews and raisins

Dinner: Spaghetti with garden greens; broccoli, green beans and courgette

3

DAY 3

EXERCISE

16-Minute Inch-Loss Walk (see page 59)

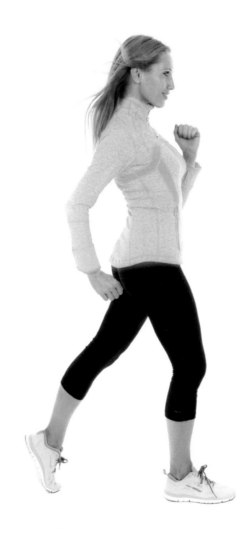

MENU

Breakfast: Mashed avocado on toasted rye bread

Snack: Carrot sticks dipped in a small amount of cottage cheese

Lunch: Half a jacket potato with sweet corn and wafer-thin ham

Snack: Low-fat yoghurt with added sprinkling of sunflower seeds

Dinner: Honey- and ginger-glazed salmon with hazelnut and cucumber; tomato and chive salad

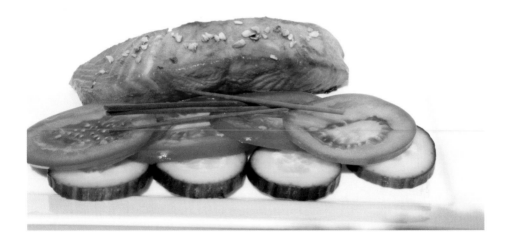

DAY 4

EXERCISE

Total-body move: Reach for the Stars Lunge. Complete 20 reps each leg.

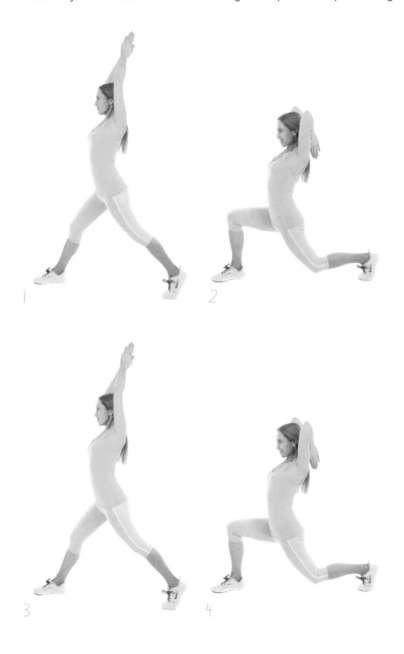

MENU

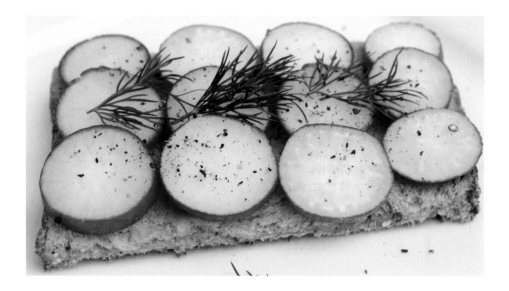

Breakfast: Porridge with added pear slices and sunflower seeds

Snack: Half a slice of toast topped with a thin layer of low-fat cream cheese and sliced radish with dill

Lunch: Bowl of tomato and basil soup with wholemeal pita bread

Snack: Banana and handful of raisins

Dinner: Lean mince with courgette spaghetti—make normal spaghetti mince, but swap spaghetti for courgette noodles. Use a spiralizer or finely grate courgette, and then fry in a 1-cal oil spray for a couple of minutes on a medium heat. It tastes just like pasta.

DAY 5

EXERCISE

16-Minute Inch-Loss Walk (see page 59)

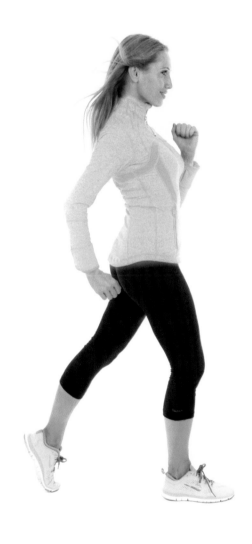

MENU

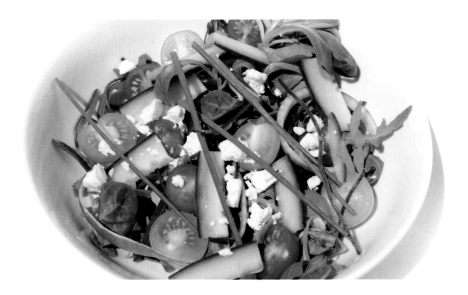

Breakfast: Avocado and tomato on wholegrain toast

Snack: Cucumber sticks wrapped in three turkey slices

Lunch: Feta cheese with cherry tomatoes and sliced red onion with a drizzle of balsamic vinegar

Snack: Handful of grapes and a few pecan nuts

Dinner: Grilled cod fillet with a drizzle of lime and served with ratatouille

3

DAY 6

EXERCISE

Total-body move: Reach for the Stars Lunge. Complete 30 reps each leg.

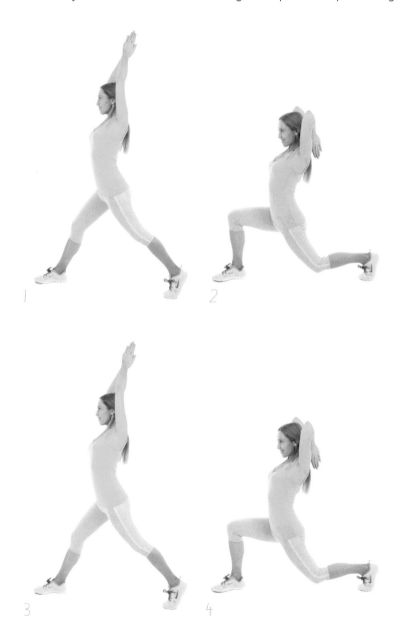

MENU

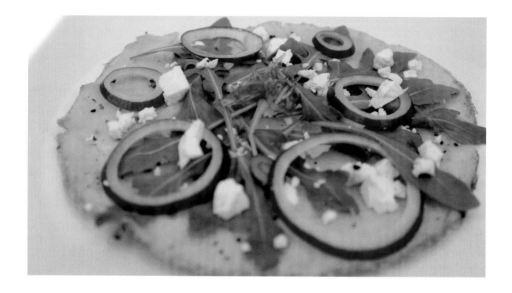

Breakfast: Banana, sultanas and honey mixed in with natural yoghurt

Snack: Cherry tomatoes with cottage cheese

Lunch: Rocket with red onion and feta omelette

Snack: Pear with handful of sunflower seeds

Dinner: Grilled chicken breast with peas and sweet potato mash

DAY 7

DAY OFF!

Now it's time to look back and reflect on how well you have done. Today is a pamper day.

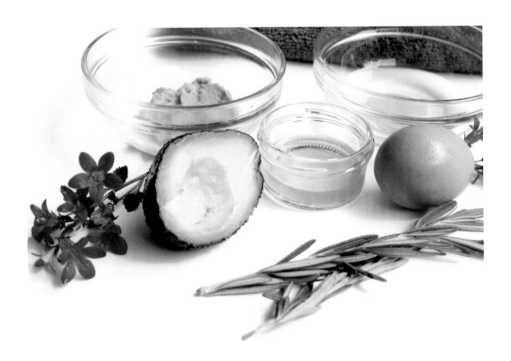

PAMPER TREAT

Homemade Nourishing Hair Mask

What you need:

Avocado
1 egg
Small amount of olive oil

First mash up your avocado into a fine creamy paste (you only need to use half). Then whisk the egg. Place the whisked egg into the avocado paste, and then drizzle a little oil. Mix thoroughly together. Apply this mixture to your wet hair just after washing it. Pin up your hair and leave in for about 10 minutes. Then rinse off hair mask with COLD water (never hot). Be sure to rinse thoroughly. The three ingredients in this hair mask help penetrate the hair follicles and will leave your hair shiny and soft.

RESULTS

Today you can also redo your measurements, and if you have time, quickly redo your 0.5 walk test and see what time you do it in.

3

MENU

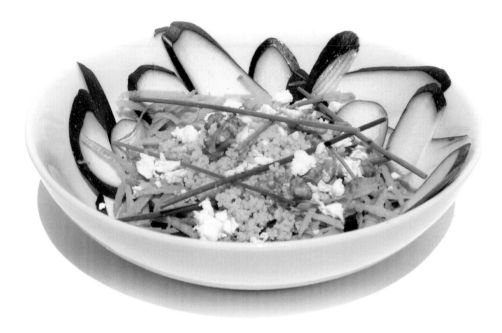

Breakfast: Poached egg on a wholemeal muffin

Snack: Banana

Lunch: Bowl of cous cous with grated carrot, sliced courgettes, crumbled feta and crushed walnuts

Snack: Oatcake with peanut butter

Dinner: Chicken and vegetables served on a heated wholemeal tortilla

SUMMARY FOR WEEK 1

Well done for completing this week. You will already be feeling so many benefits from this. Your waistband will be feeling looser, you will have more energy and you will be looking forward to starting week 2, which is going to bring you even more results.

Write a note to yourself on how you feel.	Write down the benefits you feel from this week.

3

WEEK 2

MOTTO FOR WEEK 2:

Keep up the good work.

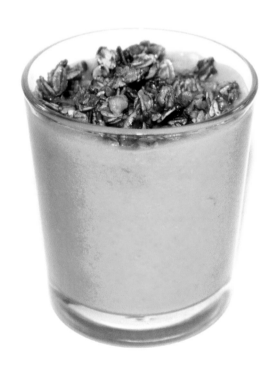

BOOTY AND AB TONER WALKING WORKOUT

Booty and Ab Toner Walk:

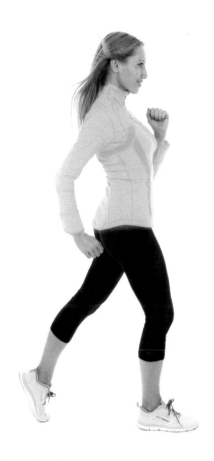

Time	Walk style (see page 29)	Intensity (see page 34)
1:30 minutes	Brisk Walk	5
1 minute	Ab Toning Stride	5.5
1 minute	Deeper Stride	6
30 seconds	Arms Crossed Stride	6
Repeat this sequence 4 times.		

3

TOTAL-BODY TONER FOR WEEK 2: ANGEL SWEEP

This total-body move is called the **Angel Sweep**, named by @joackling on Instagram.

This sideways stepping move tones and sculpts your inner and outer thighs, lifts your bottom, tightens your abs and shapes and slims your arms and shoulders.

How to do it:

- Stand with your feet together, and drop into a slight squat position so that your knees are bent and both arms fully extended forwards with your palms facing up.
- Sink slightly deeper into your squat. At the same time open your arms to the side so that your hands are in line with your shoulders.
- Lunge one foot out to the side, and then bring your opposite hand towards the inside of the foot, while simultaneously lifting the other arm out high behind you.
- Push back up to your squat with arms wide open.
- Come up to the starting position by bringing both arms back to the centre.
- Now sink slightly deeper into your squat and again open your arms so that your hands are in line with your shoulders.
- Lunge the other foot out to the side, and then bring your opposite hand towards the inside of the foot, while simultaneously lifting the other arm out high behind you.

This is the whole move. I will set you different amounts of repetitions for this move as we progress through week 2.

(For instructions on how to do the **Angel Sweep** exercise, watch the video "How to do the Angel Sweep" on my YouTube channel.)

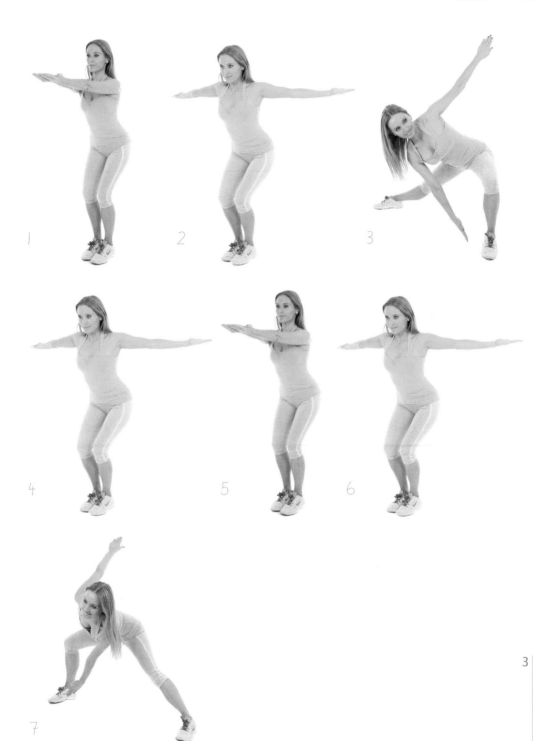

DAY 8

EXERCISE

Booty and Ab Toner Walk (see page 79)

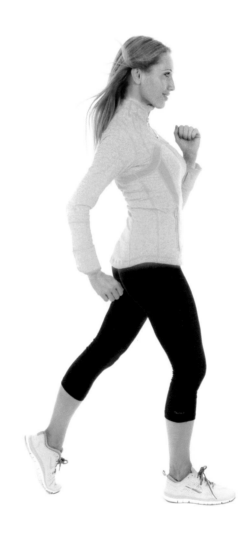

MENU

Breakfast: Low-fat plain Greek yoghurt with 1 tablespoon of cocoa powder and a pinch of cinnamon

Snack: 1 banana and a few raisins

Lunch: Half of an avocado (you will use the other half tomorrow), peas and parmesan with grated orange zest as an open, wholemeal sandwich

Snack: Carrot sticks with a small amount of hummus

Dinner: Grilled chicken breast with steamed asparagus and mixed green salad

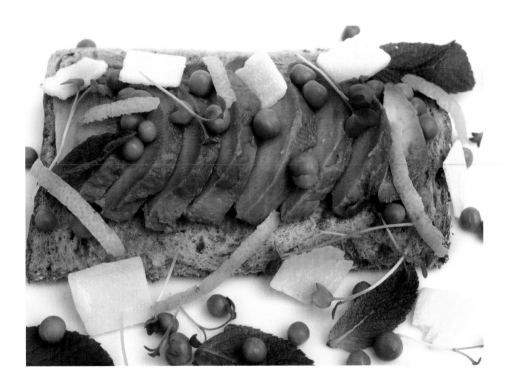

DAY 9

EXERCISE

Total-body move: Angel Sweep. Complete 10 reps.

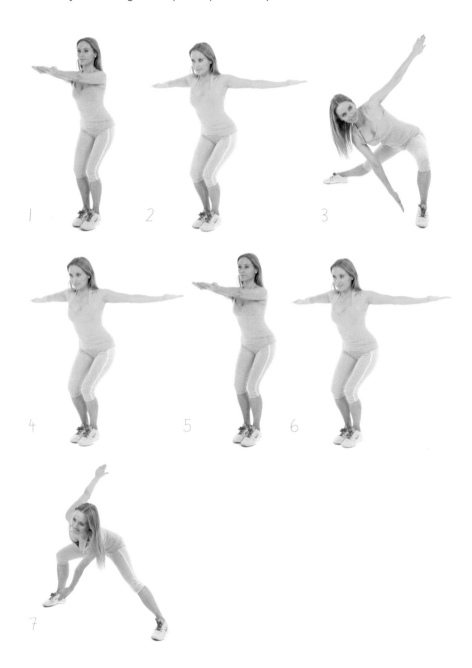

MENU

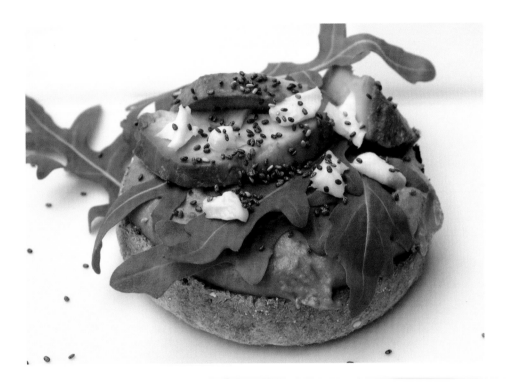

Breakfast: Small bowl of whole-grain cereal with semi-skimmed milk and chopped banana

Snack: Two small squares of dark chocolate

Lunch: Toasted wholemeal muffin with beetroot mixed with quark (low-fat cream cheese), topped with rocket, half an avocado, crumbled feta and poppy seeds

Snack: Small handful of cashews and raisins

Dinner: Half of a sweet jacket potato with tuna, sweet corn and chopped spring onion

3

DAY 10

EXERCISE

Booty and Ab Toner Walk (see page 79)

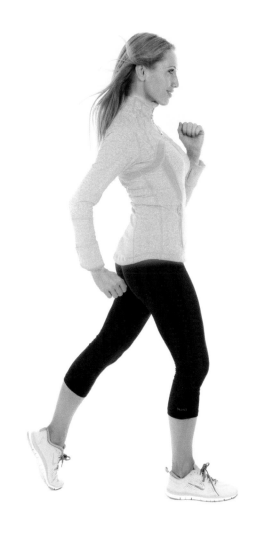

MENU

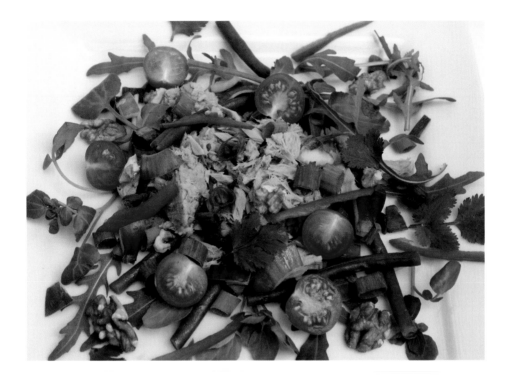

Breakfast: Scrambled eggs on wholemeal toast, topped with a sprinkle of poppy seeds

Snack: Raw broccoli florets dipped in cottage cheese

Lunch: Tuna, tomato and mixed salad

Snack: Low-fat yoghurt with a small amount of added oats

Dinner: Pasta with grilled asparagus and mushrooms, topped with grated parmesan and orange zest

DAY 11

EXERCISE

Total-body move: Angel Sweep. Complete 16 reps.

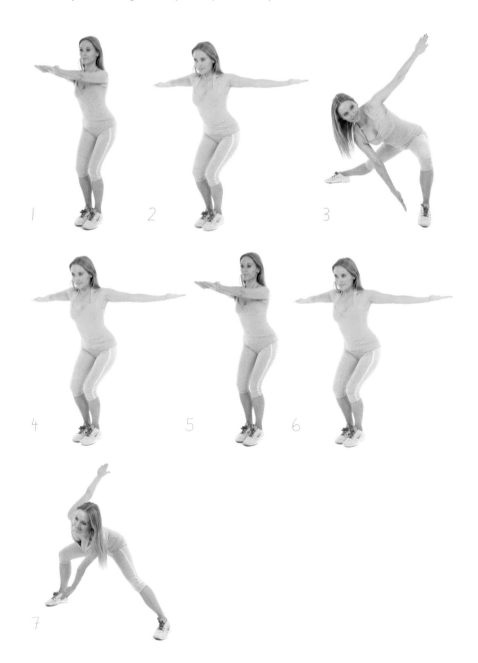

MENU

Breakfast: Porridge with added kiwi and a couple of crushed pecans

Snack: Strawberry slices with cottage cheese

Lunch: Bowl of low-fat vegetable soup and an oatcake

Snack: Banana and a handful of raisins

Dinner: Grilled salmon fillet on brown rice with Greek yoghurt and dill dressing with lime

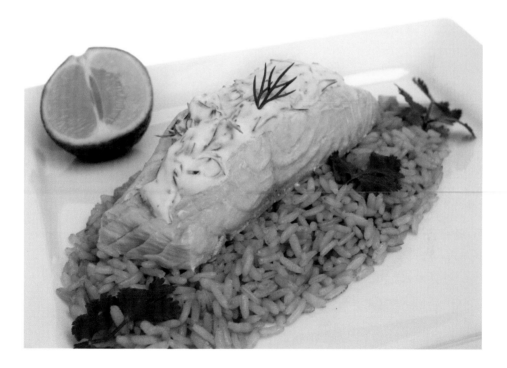

DAY 12

EXERCISE

Booty and Ab Toner Walk (see page 79)

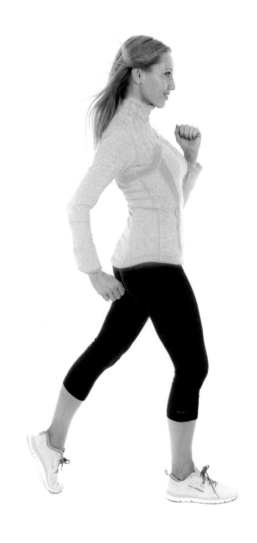

MENU

Breakfast: Apple crumble (Prepare the night before: Wash, core and slice the apple. Then boil the apple in a pan until it is cooked. Drain the pan, and mash the apple or place in a blender. Let it cool and put it in the fridge overnight. In the morning, heat the apple and top with porridge oats and a sprinkle of cinnamon.)

Snack: Cucumber sticks wrapped in wafer-thin ham slices

Lunch: Chicken wholemeal tortilla wrap with grated carrot, cucumber and chopped spring onions and a small amount of low-fat Greek yoghurt

Snack: 2 small squares of dark chocolate

Dinner: Spaghetti Bolognese with courgette noodles

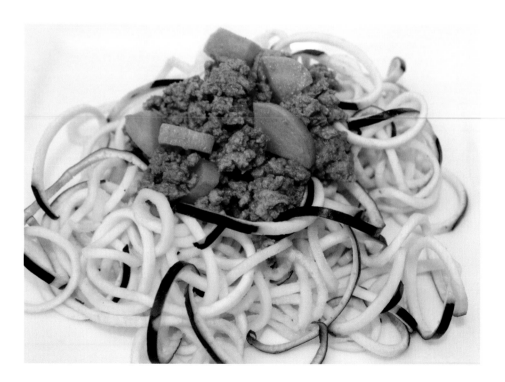

3

DAY 13

EXERCISE

Total-body move: Angel Sweep. Complete 20 reps.

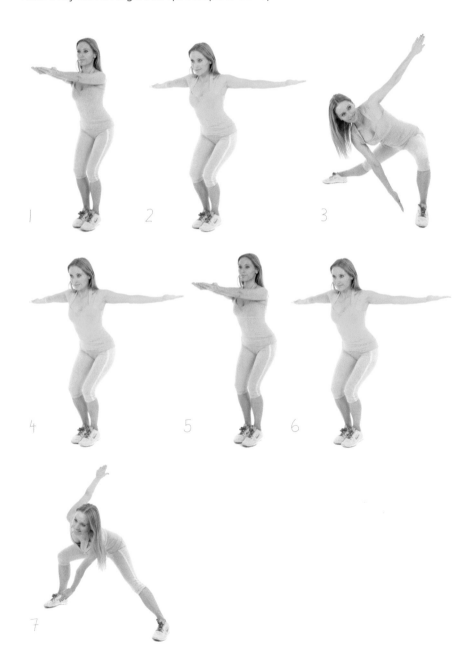

MENU

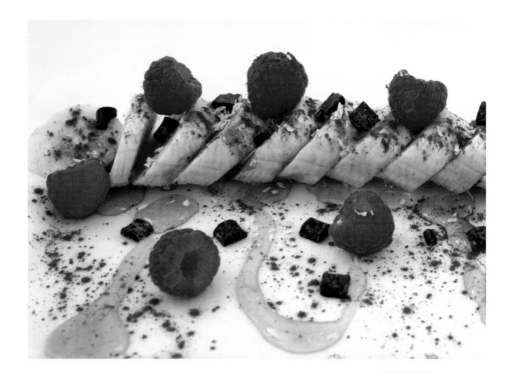

Breakfast: Banana split (Sliced banana with added raspberries, 1 square of dark chocolate finely grated, sprinkle of coconut, drizzle of honey and pinch of cinnamon)

Snack: Mashed avocado on a rice cake

Lunch: Wholemeal tuna salad with rocket and red onion sandwich

Snack: Small piece of cheese with apple slices

Dinner: Grilled fillet steak with green salad

3

DAY 14

DAY OFF!

Time to look back and reflect on how well you have done. Today is also a pamper day.

PAMPER TREAT

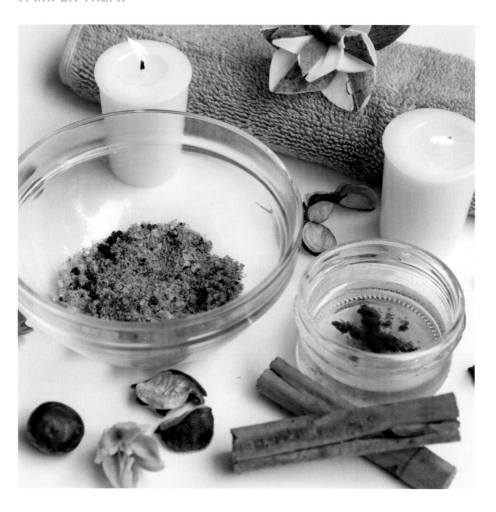

CINAMMON SUGAR SOUFFLÉ BODY MIX

Buff up your skin with my cinnamon sugar soufflé body mix.

What you need:

1 tablespoon of rolled oats

3 tablespoons of olive oil

2 tablespoons of sugar

A big pinch of cinnamon

Mix all the ingredients together into a bowl. Apply this mixture all over your body when you are in the bath or shower. The oats and the sugar help to remove any dead skin cells; the oil helps lock in moisture; and the cinnamon makes it smell divine. Leave on your skin for at least 10 minutes, and then thoroughly rinse it off.

Firmly pat your skin dry with a towel.

RESULTS

Today you can also redo your measurements, and, if you have time, quickly redo your Walk Fit test and see what time you do it in.

3

MENU

Breakfast: Banana and cinnamon omelette (Make your normal omelette mix then add in very finely sliced banana pieces and a pinch of cinnamon powder. Cook your omelette as normal. Then in a small frying pan, add a little low-cal spray oil. Brown the banana slightly, and pour over your omelette mix. Cook normally. Then flip to cook the other side. Once cooked, sprinkle on a little cinnamon.)

Snack: Pecans and grapes

Lunch: Turkey salad with red onion, rocket and black olives on wholemeal pita

Snack: Oatcake with peanut butter

Dinner: Poached salmon with courgettes spirals and spring onion salad

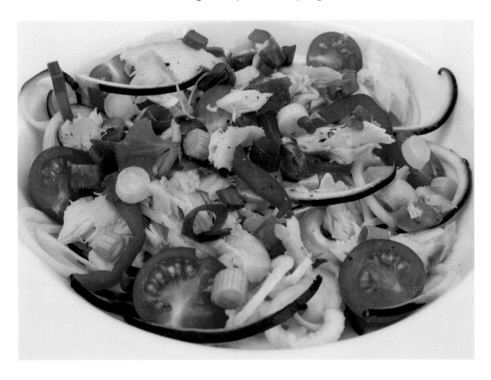

SUMMARY FOR WEEK 2

Well done for completing this week. You will already be feeling so many benefits from this and also will now have heaps of energy to get going on week 3.

Write a note to yourself here on how you feel.	Write down the benefits you feel from this week.

WEEK 3

Motto for Week 3

> ## You are close to reaching your goal.

16-MINUTE FAT-BURNING WALKING WORKOUT

16-Minute Fat-Burning Walk

Time	Walk style (see page 29)	Intensity (see page 34)
1 minute	Brisk Walk	5.5
1 minute	Ab Toning Stride	6.0
1 minute	Faster Walk	6.5
30 seconds	Even Faster Walk	6.75
30 seconds	Brisk Walk	
Repeat this sequence 4 times.		

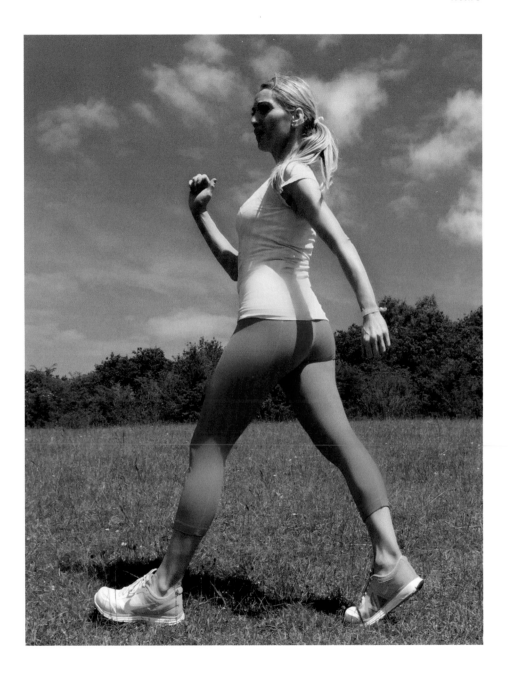

TOTAL-BODY TONER FOR WEEK 3: WALK IT OUT WAIST TONER

This total-body move is called the **Walk it Out Waist Toner**, and it was named by @hattiwr.s on Instagram.

This move tones your legs, waist, bottom, abs, chest and arms, meaning you are going to be toning all over. This move also helps improve your flexibility and supercharge your calorie burn because you are engaging so many muscles.

How to do it:

- Start by standing with good, upright posture.
- Start to squat while simultaneously walking your hands down your legs.
- Place both hands on the floor.
- Walk out both hands so that you are in a full plank with arms extended.
- Bend one leg and bring it under your body as if you are trying to get that knee to touch your opposite elbow. Then bring that leg back into the plank position and repeat on the opposite leg.
- From the plank, walk yourself back up to the starting position.

You can see the full instruction video "How to do the Walk It Out Waist Toner" on my YouTube Channel.

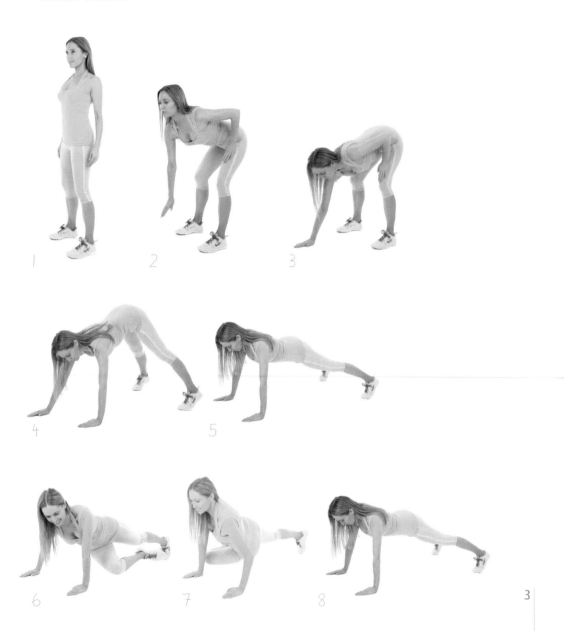

3

DAY 15

EXERCISE

16-Minute Fat-Burning Walk (see page 98)

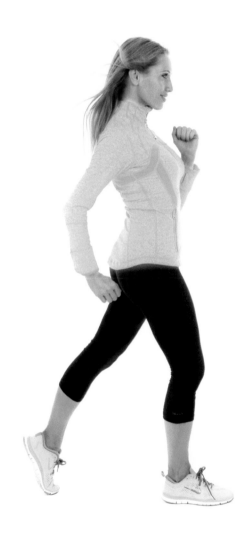

MENU

Breakfast: Scrambled eggs with an avocado

Snack: Fruit smoothie

Lunch: Tuna and mozzarella on mixed bean salad with red onion and sliced green pepper

Snack: Raisins and cashews

Dinner: Grilled aubergine slices with natural Greek yoghurt with added pomegranates, served on salad leaves

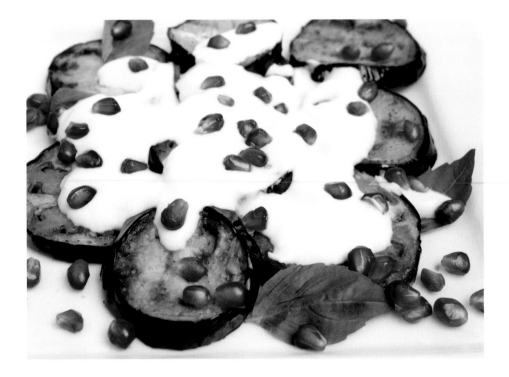

DAY 16

EXERCISE

Total-body move: Walk it Out Waist Toner. Complete 6 reps.

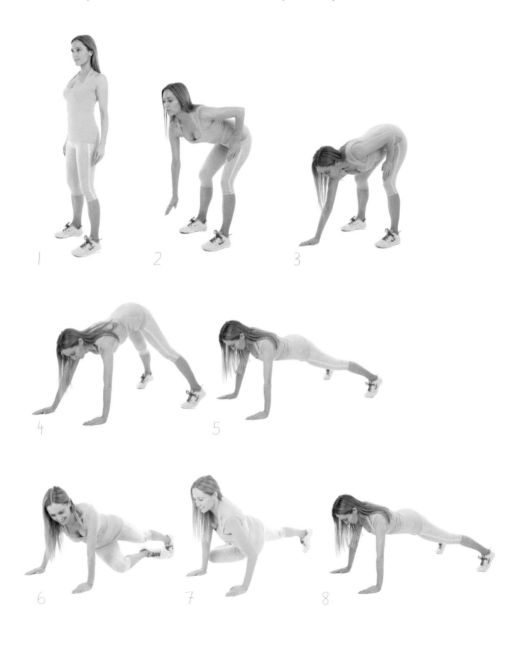

MENU

Breakfast: Greek yoghurt with kiwi and pomegranate

Snack: Carrot and hummus

Lunch: Wholemeal pita stuffed with grated carrot, grated red cabbage and turkey slices

Snack: Dates cut open with a little peanut butter

Dinner: Prawn and pea wholemeal stir-fry

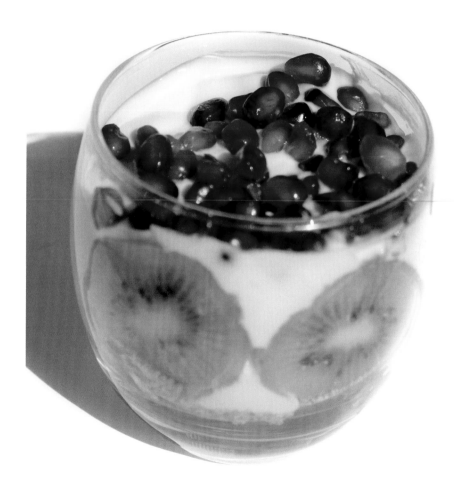

3

DAY 17

EXERCISE

16-Minute Fat-Burning Walk (see page 98)

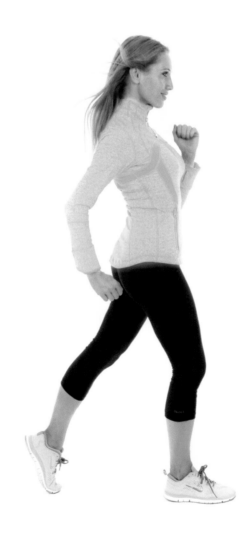

MENU

Breakfast: Whole-grain cereal topped with banana and raisins

Snack: Hummus on a rice cake

Lunch: Half a sweet jacket potato with cottage cheese and spring onion

Snack: Pear with pecans

Dinner: Courgette mini pizza (Cut your courgette into quarter-inch thick round sections. Then boil the sections in a saucepan for a couple of minutes, drain and add a very small amount of tomato puree—preferably a no-sugar one, if possible. Then sprinkle some grated mozzarella, herbs and spices over the courgette chunks. Place under a grill on a medium heat until golden brown.)

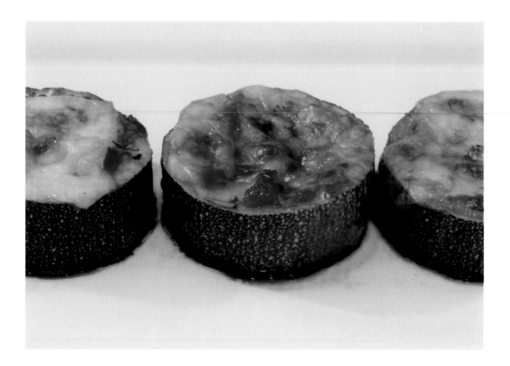

3

DAY 18

EXERCISE

Total-body move: Walk it Out Waist Toner. Complete 10 reps.

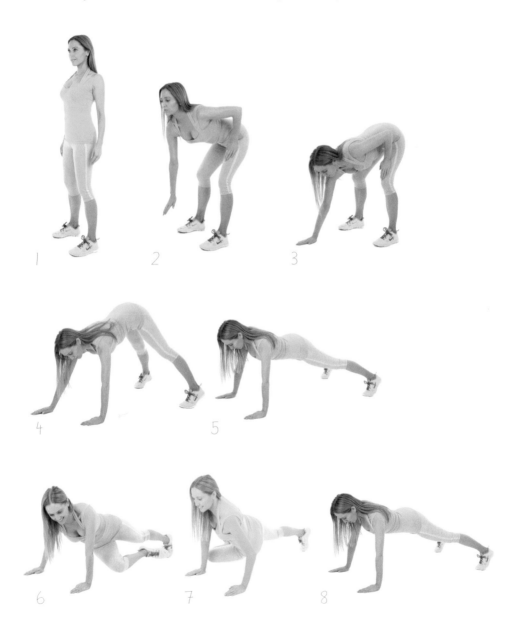

MENU

Breakfast: Wholemeal toast with thinly spread peanut butter and small pineapple chunks

Snack: Banana and raisins

Lunch: Avocado and tuna salad with rocket and chopped red pepper

Snack: Latté and pecans

Dinner: Lemon-drizzled grilled chicken breast with rocket, feta salad and orange peel zest

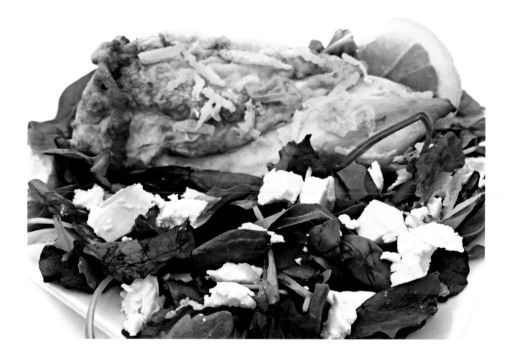

DAY 19

EXERCISE

16-Minute Fat-Burning Walk (see page 98)

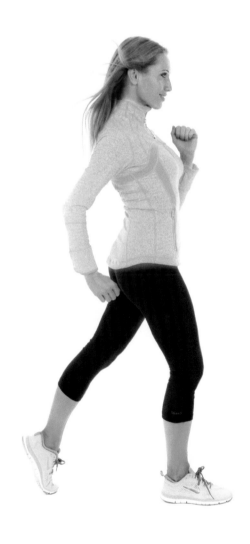

MENU

Breakfast: Strawberry and hazelnut crumble smoothie (In a blender, add a small amount of low-fat natural yoghurt, 5 washed and chopped strawberries and a couple of hazelnuts. Blend, pour into a glass and top with a handful of porridge oats.)

Snack: 2 thin turkey slices with cherry tomatoes

Lunch: Tuna, tomatoes, green beans, red pepper and rocket salad

Dinner: Vegetable stir-fry with thinly sliced strips of fillet beef

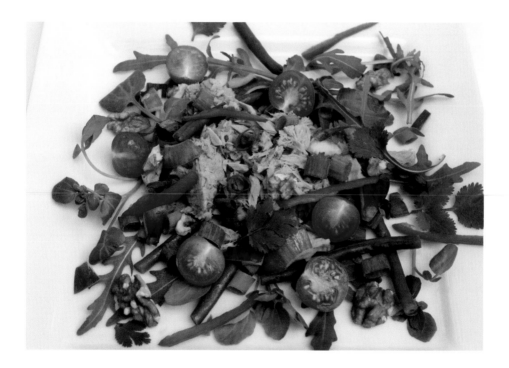

DAY 20

EXERCISE

Total-body move: Walk it Out Waist Toner. Complete 12 reps.

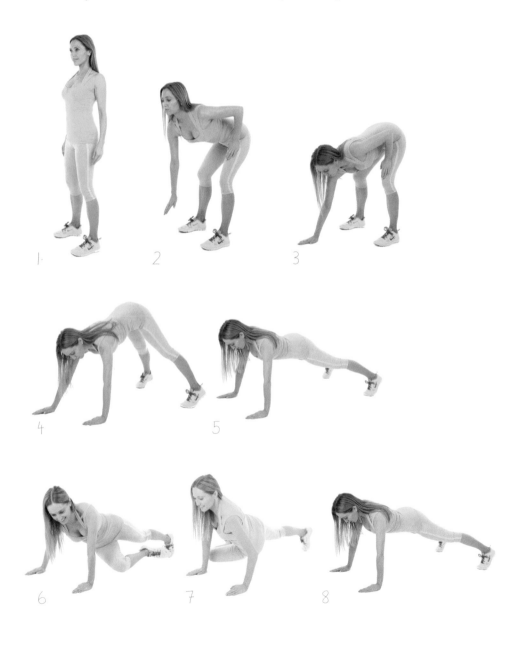

MENU

Breakfast: Poached egg on a wholemeal muffin, topped with a little low-fat Greek yoghurt and poppy seeds

Snack: Banana and a few almonds

Lunch: Half a sweet potato with tuna and chopped red pepper

Snack: Latté and two *small* squares of dark chocolate

Dinner: Avocado with grilled asparagus, pomegranate and feta salad

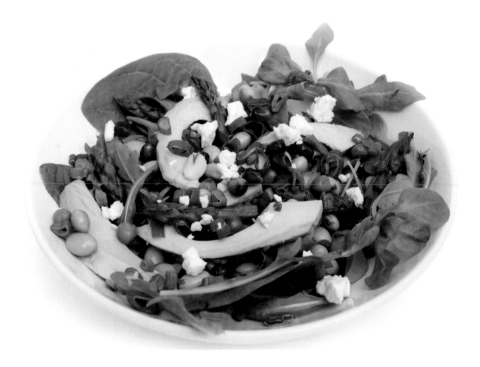

4

DAY 21

DAY OFF!

Time to look back and reflect on how well you have done over the past weeks. Today is also a pamper day.

PAMPER TREAT

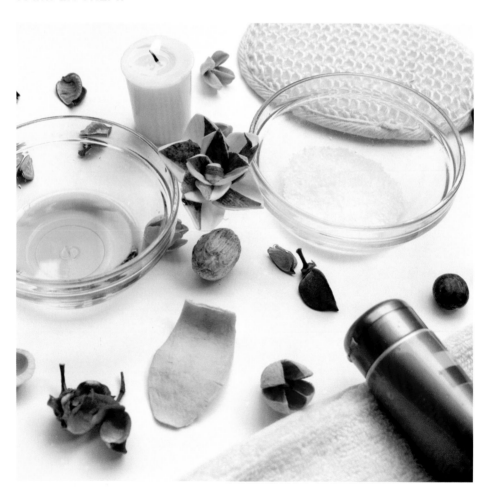

MAKEOVER BODY GLOW

If you want to do an "after" photo from all your training for the last 21 days, then why not do this pamper treat so that tomorrow you will have a healthy golden glow when you take your "after" photo. You can always keep that on hand as your own personal motivation.

What you need:

1 tablespoon oil

2 tablespoons rock salt

Self-tanning lotion

Mix the oil and rock salt together in a bowl. Apply this mixture all over your body when you are in the bath or the shower. Leave on your skin for at least 5 minutes, and then thoroughly rinse off. Be sure to firmly pat your skin dry with a towel and absorb any excess oil. Then apply your self-tanning lotion. Tomorrow you will wake up with a beautiful glow and a new super fit and healthy body, ready to take your selfie.

RESULTS

Today you can also redo your measurements. Now you should see such a difference. Refer back to week 1 to see how well you have done. Also, redo your Walk Fit test and see how much faster you now complete this.

4

MENU

Breakfast: Banana Pancakes with Peanut Butter and Strawberries. Whisk 1 egg and mash up a banana into a creamy paste. Mix the banana paste and egg together in a pan on a medium heat. Use a couple of sprays of 1-cal spray oil, and pour in half your mixture (this is perfect for 1 small pancake) into a skillet and cook both sides for a minute or so, or until golden. Then cook the rest of your mixture the same way. Or, if you prefer, cook the whole mixture for one large pancake. Spread on a little peanut butter and top with your strawberries.

(I left the best till last; this is my absolute favourite. And, if you use social media and want to share your pictures of your healthy foods with me, please do, using this hashtag: #lucyhealthyfood.)

Snack: Cherry tomatoes and a little cottage cheese

Lunch: Grated courgette, chicken breast, chopped spring onions, a dollop of natural Greek yoghurt and squeezed fresh lime

Snack: Peach and a few almonds

Dinner: Grilled white fish with lemon, olive oil and herbs with roasted cherry tomatoes and asparagus

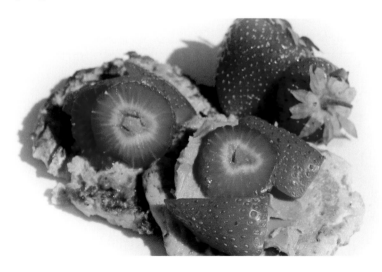

SUMMARY FOR WEEK 3

Well done for completing this 21-day plan. You will have noticed the inches have dropped off, and your body will feel tighter and more defined. You will have turned back your body clock by lifting certain areas that can head south without exercise. More importantly, you will be feeling so much fitter and more energetic, and, most importantly, you will have improved your health and wellbeing.

Write a note to yourself here on how you feel.	Write down the benefits you feel from completing the 21-day plan.

4

Part 4

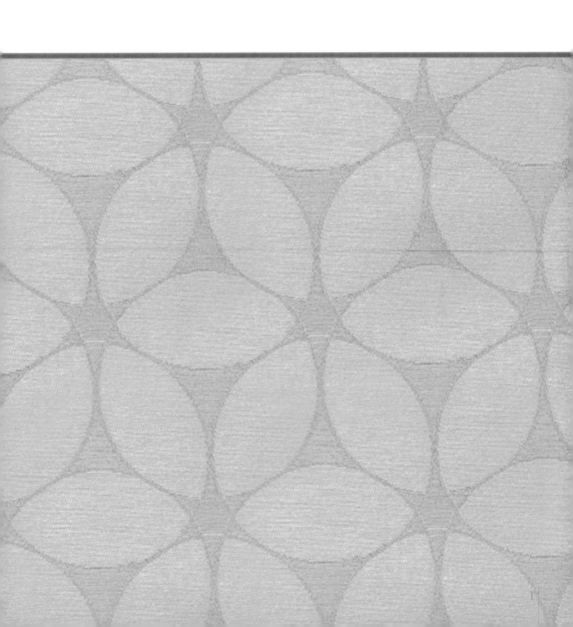

Part 4

HOW TO MAINTAIN YOUR
NEW WEIGHT LOSS

You are now going to be feeling and looking great, and you obviously want to keep feeling this good, having energy and looking years younger.

In the last 21 days (by the way, I write all my fitness and weight-loss plans in this timeframe as this is all it takes to see results and for the body and mind to adjust and feel comfortable with these new healthy habits), you will have got used to this active lifestyle. I bet you any money that if I said, okay, now eat processed, unhealthy foods and do no exercise, you would say, no way! For me, this is so exciting because you are now set to be healthy for life.

To maintain your healthy lifestyle now is very easy. What you should do is aim to complete three to four walks a week, and this book presents three different styles you can choose. Then for your body toning, here is a new circuit in which you do all three moves that you have become familiar with over the last 21 days. Because you are now super fit, let's add them all together.

MAINTENCE MAKEOVER ROUTINE

Exercise 1: Reach for the Stars Lunge (see page 60)

Repetitions: 5 reps each leg

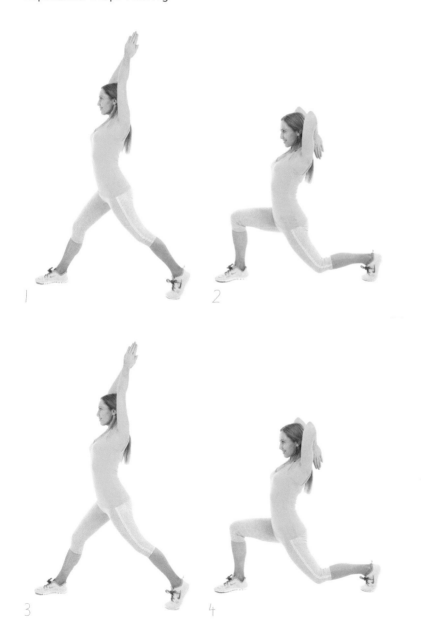

4

Exercise 2: Angel Sweep (see page 80)

Repetitions: 5 reps

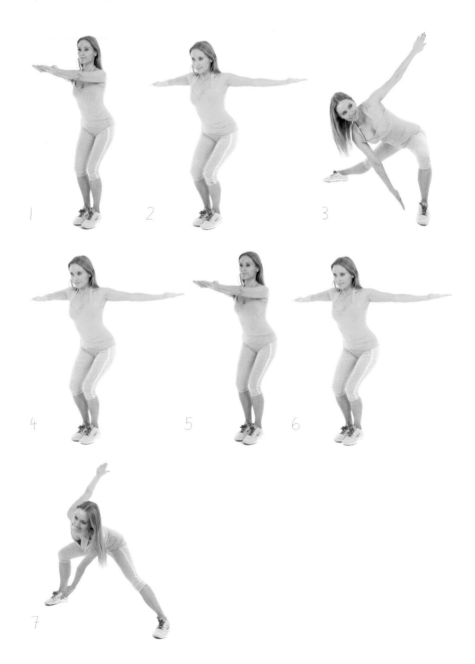

Exercise 3: Walk It Out Waist Toner (see page 100)

Repetitions: 5 reps

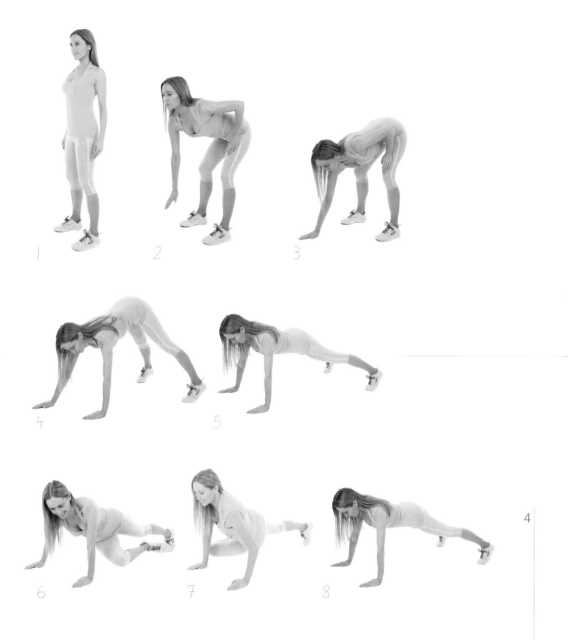

4

Sample Weekly Schedule

Monday	Tuesday	Wednesday	Thursday	Friday	Saturday	Sunday
Booty and Ab Toner Walk	Maintenance Makeover Routine	16-Minute Inch-Loss Walk	Maintenance Makeover Routine	16-Minute Fat-Burning Walk	Workout video from Lucy's YouTube Channel: LWR Fitness Channel	Pamper day

Tip: For the Maintenance Makeover Routine, you can always add a few more reps if you want to increase the difficulty. Remember to perform these three exercises slowly, and put 100 per cent focus into what you are doing. Also, I have a huge selection of home fitness videos on my YouTube Channel which you could subscribe to: LWRFitness Channel

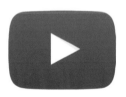

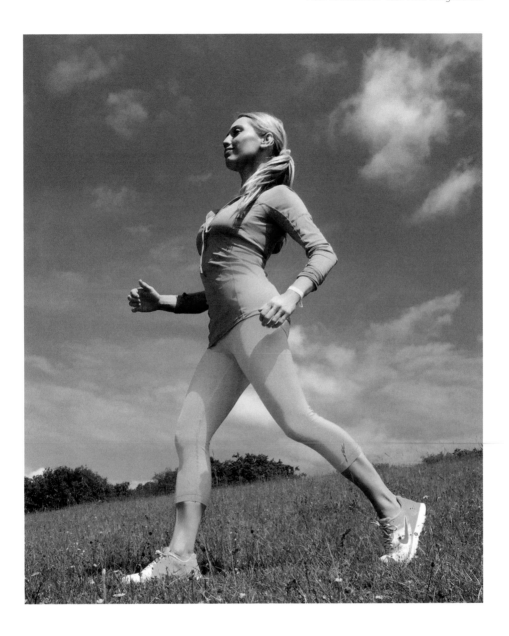

EAT YOURSELF YOUNGER

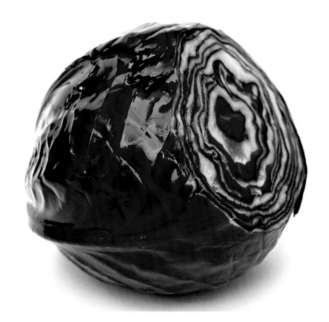

Eat right, Look younger

By making the right food choices you can help make yourself look younger. Eating right is the best way to slow down the aging process. It gives you a healthy glow and plenty of energy, not to mention keeps you in tip-top shape.

Nature really does provide us with everything we need, and when it comes to keeping ourselves in good condition, the food we eat can be much more effective than spending a fortune on things like expensive face creams which only affect the outer layers of the skin. What is more important is feeding the skin from the inside out, so it is true to say you really can eat yourself younger and fitter.

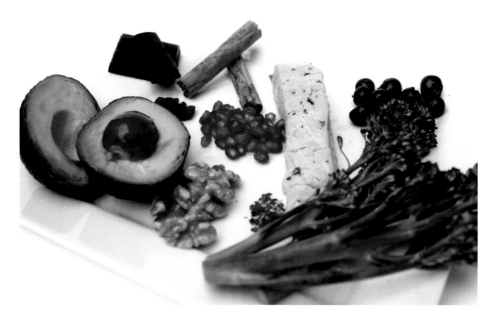

When it comes to anti-aging foods we are spoilt for choice, as there are so many of them. I am going to list my top 10 and show you some healthy, anti-aging recipes and snacks that you can create with these foods.

First, let's look at what essential anti-aging foods should be in our shopping basket.

4

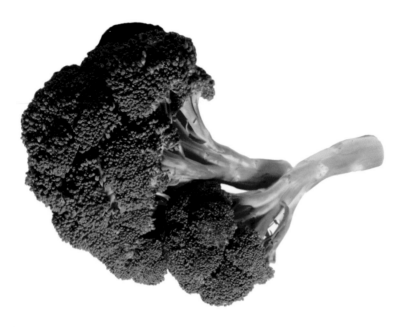

1. **Broccoli**

   This vibrant green vegetable has a big dose of vitamin C, which helps to keep the skin clear. Broccoli also has nutrients that help the liver with detoxification.

2. **Avocado**

   These delicious, creamy green fruits are very high in omega-9 fatty acid, which is what helps our skin retain moisture. This keeps your skin plumped and supple.

3. **Walnuts**

   These nuts are winners for you hair, giving you a glossy mane! They have a high abundance of omega-3 fatty acids, which help keep your hair hydrated. They also have a large amount of vitamin E, which helps repair damaged follicles, so eat your walnuts and have a good hair day, every day.

4. **Salmon**

   This is definitely worth featuring as a catch of the day, as EPA (eicosapentaenoic acid) can be found in this oily fish. This is great for helping to preserve collagen fibre, meaning you get smoother skin and fewer wrinkles.

5. **Blueberries**

These berries may be small, but don't be fooled. They have a powerful punch of antioxidants in them, and the darker they are, the more powerful they are. These help to protect the skin from aging.

6. **Pomegranates**

The crimson little budlike seeds found in pomegranates are a very high source of vitamins C and K, and they're high in minerals, which are responsible for keeping our skin looking clear and smooth.

7. **Red cabbage**

This vibrantly coloured cabbage is a rich source of sulphur. This is a mineral that can help reduce inflammation in the skin. It is also high in vitamin E, which is great for keeping your skin glowing.

8. **Watermelon**

The clue is in the name: This superfruit is mostly water, which makes it super hydrating. It keeps your skin fully hydrated from inside out and diminishes any fine lines.

9. **Sweet potatoes**

These definitely deserve to be called sweet as they do wonders for our skin. They contain beta-carotene, which is an antioxidant that looks after our skin, eyes, and bones.

10. **Dark chocolate**

Yes, you read that right. Dark chocolate is good for us. You need to find one that is high in cocoa content, because cocoa has nutrients in it that can help increase the blood flow to our skin, thus helping to keep our skin cells working at full capacity.

ANTI-AGING RECIPES

LUSCIOUS LIME AND AVOCADO PURÉE STUFFED RED SLIPPER

This tasty snack—or it could also be a light lunch—will give your skin the same glow that you get from having a facial.

Ingredients

1 sweet red pepper

1 avocado

Small amount of feta

1 lime

Several coriander leaves

Small red chilli pepper

Instructions

Wash your sweet red pepper and cut it open. Scoop out the seeds, preparing this as your edible base.

Peel and remove the stone from the avocado. Place in a blender and add a generous squeeze of fresh lime and a few washed coriander leaves. Blend until mixture has a creamy texture, and then pour the lime and avocado purée into your pepper. Finally, top with some crumbled feta and finely chopped chilli pepper.

Depending on taste, you can either leave out the chilli pepper seeds, or, if you like the extra hot kick, keep them in.

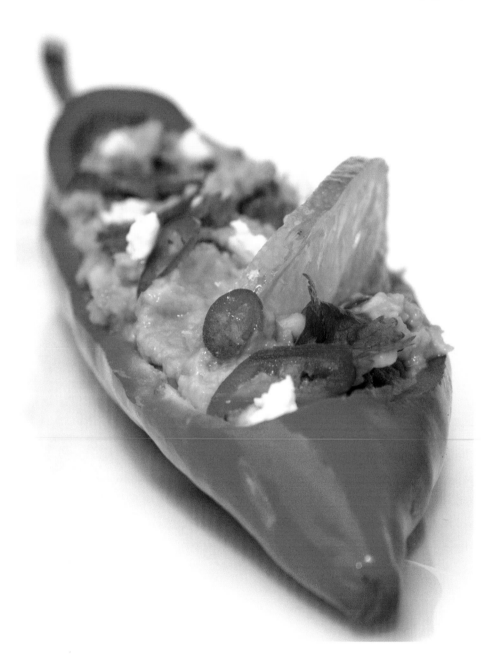

4

QUICK CRUNCHY COLESLAW

This is super delicious and has so many anti-aging ingredients that it will make you look as radiant as the dish itself.

Ingredients

1/4 red cabbage

1 carrot

1 apple

Handful of raisins

Several pumpkin seeds

2 tablespoons of low-fat natural yoghurt

1 celery stick

Instructions

Wash your cabbage and peel off the outer leaf. I use a leaf or two to serve the coleslaw in, so keep a couple spares. Finely chop the cabbage. Then wash the carrot, apple and celery and finely slice these. Put the low-fat natural yoghurt into a bowl, add all the ingredients, and mix together. That is your crunchy coleslaw, which you can serve in your red cabbage leaves. It tastes as good as it looks.

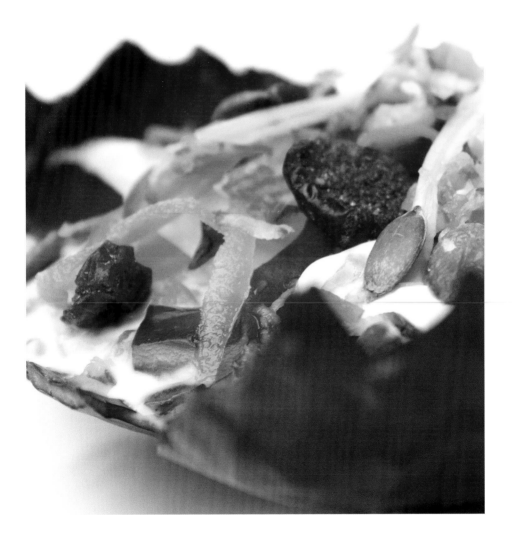

SWEET POTATO AND RED KIDNEY BEAN BURGER

This burger is just oozing with goodness, and the sweet potato and kidney beans will keep your skin plumped and radiant.

Ingredients

1 sweet potato

1 small tin of cooked kidney beans

Half a slice of wholemeal bread

2 spring onions

Crisp lettuce leaf

Red onion

Cherry tomatoes

Seasoning

Instructions

Preheat oven to medium heat. Place half a slice of wholemeal bread in a blender and blend to create breadcrumbs, and then place breadcrumbs on a baking tray. Lay them out evenly and spray just a couple of squirts of a low-calorie, good quality oil. Then place the baking tray in the centre of the oven and bake for about 20 minutes or until golden, stirring them halfway through baking. Peel and chop the sweet potato. Heat a pan of boiling water, and then add in the sweet potato. Cook for about 15 to 20 minutes on medium heat until they are soft, and then remove from heat and drain them. Put the sweet potato and cooked kidney beans into a blender, along with washed and finely chopped spring onions, and blend together. Remove the breadcrumbs from the oven and set aside to cool. Then remove the sweet potato mixture from the blender, and on a plate, shape it into a round patty. Place onto the breadcrumbs, rolling it on both sides. Heat a frying pan on a medium heat with a little low-fat, good quality oil, and cook your sweet potato and kidney bean burger for about 3 to 4 minutes on either side until crispy and golden.

Once cooked, remove and serve with crisp lettuce leaf, red onion, and cherry tomatoes.

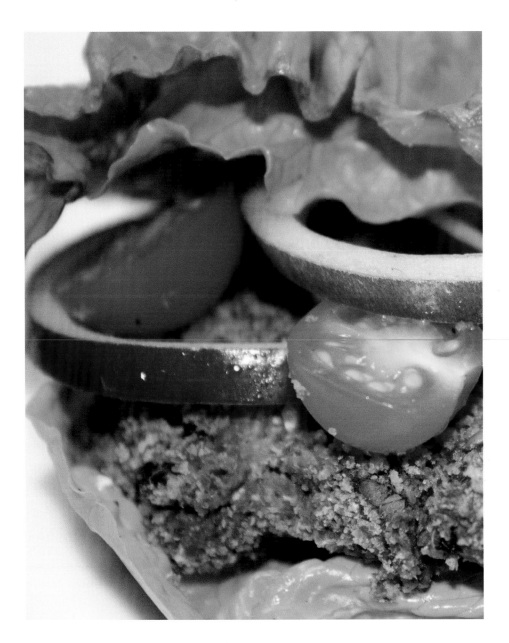

4

SUNSHINE SOUP

This soup has so many powerful ingredients high in beta-carotene that will give you a natural glow.

Ingredients

1 sweet potato

1/2 butternut squash

1 red onion

2 carrots

1 vegetable stock cube

Pinch of chilli powder

Pinch of ginger

Small amount natural Greek yoghurt

Slice of chilli

Instructions

Heat a large pan and sauté the finely sliced red onion until softened. Add the peeled and chopped sweet potato, butternut squash, and carrots, and then pour in the vegetable stock and a cup of water. Bring to a boil, and then reduce to a simmer for 20 to 25 minutes. Once cooked, remove from heat and allow to cool slightly. Then blend all the ingredients, adding your chilli and ginger powder and any extra seasoning you may require. To garnish, use finely grated carrot, a small dollop of natural Greek yoghurt, and a slice of chilli in the middle of the soup.

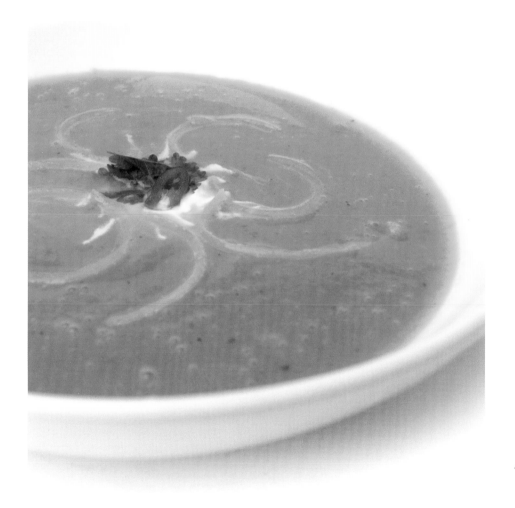

GRILLED HALLOUMI AND PEAR

This super quick salad has a delicious combination of flavours, and the texture of the halloumi works well alongside the soft, sweet pears. Topping with pomegranates gives it the nutritional benefit of youth-enhancing qualities.

Ingredients

1 pear

Small amount of halloumi

Salad leaves

Pomegranates

Instructions

Preheat your grill to medium heat. Thinly slice halloumi, and cook for about 3 minutes on both sides until golden. Wash and slice the pear. Serve up washed salad leaves on a plate, and then layer with slices of pear and halloumi and top with pomegranate seeds.

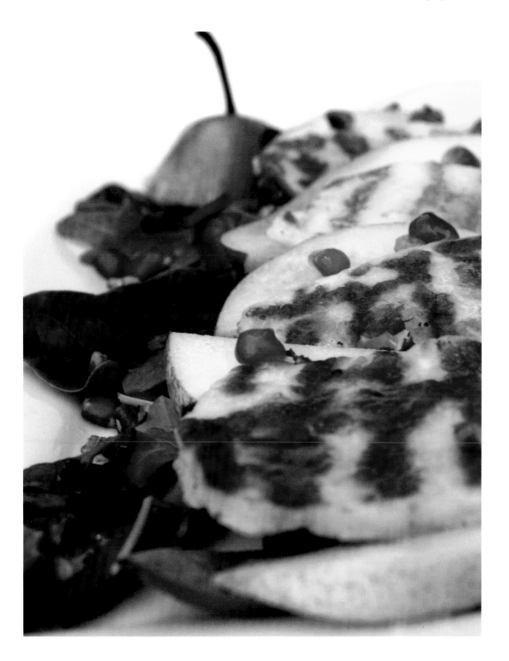

4

SUMMER SALMON, ORANGE, AND GINGER SALAD

This zesty summer salad is rich with anti-aging ingredients and very filling, so it ticks lots of boxes when it comes to having something that tastes delicious and makes you look great.

Ingredients

1 cooked salmon fillet

1 avocado

1 carrot

1 orange

1 spring onion

Pinch of ginger

Coriander leaves

Chilli flakes

Instructions

First, wash and grate your carrot into strands and place them in a bowl. Add some fresh-squeezed orange and some orange zest, plus a little sprinkling of ginger powder, and mix together. Peel and slice your avocado. On a plate, serve up your carrots and add your precooked salmon, broken into flakes, alongside your avocado. Then top with finely sliced spring onion, ripped coriander leaves, and a sprinkling of dried chilli flakes.

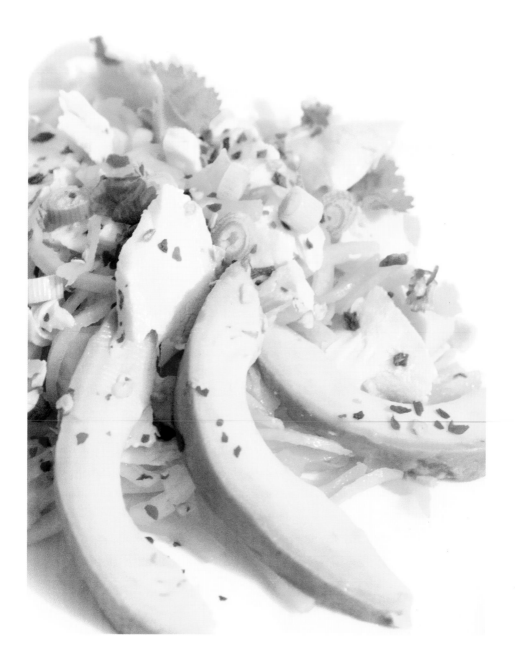

GREEN AND LEAN SALMON

This has two ingredients that are super anti-aging, so this quick dinner will help fight off those wrinkles and keep your skin plumped.

Ingredients

2 courgettes

3 broccoli florets

1 salmon fillet

Chilli flakes

Lime juice

Instructions

Preheat your oven to 180 °C (350 °F). Wrap your salmon fillet in silver foil, making a parcel with a tiny opening. Squeeze a little lime juice over the salmon and sprinkle on a few chilli flakes. Bake in the oven for about 20 minutes or until the salmon flakes away.

In the meantime, bring a saucepan of water to a boil, and cook your broccoli for about 3 to 4 minutes or until tender. Then, using a spiralizer, create your courgette noodles (or if you don't have one of these, simply grate your courgette into long strands), and then place them in a frying pan on medium heat with a couple of sprays of low-calorie oil. Cook for about 1 to 2 minutes, stirring all the time. Once cooked, remove from heat and place the courgette noodles on a plate, then add your cooked broccoli, and top with your oven-baked salmon. Finally, sprinkle on a few extra chilli flakes.

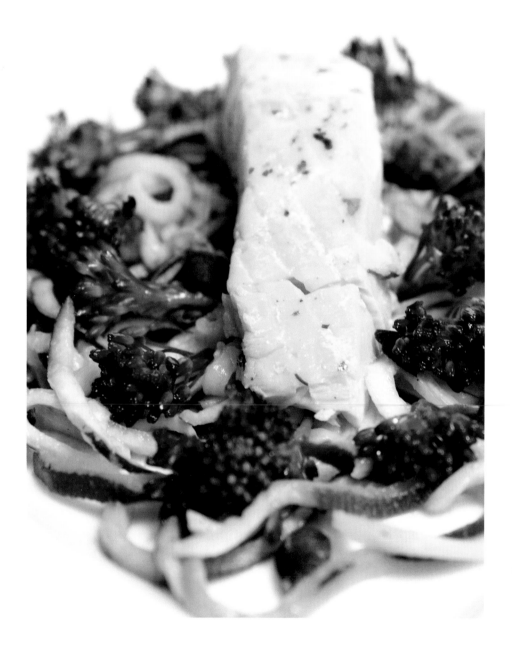

MANGO AND MAPLE ORANGE CRUNCH

This zesty pudding in a glass is a mouth-watering treat that is high in beta-carotene, which gives your skin a natural glow.

Ingredients

1 mango

1 orange

2 teaspoons maple syrup

Handful of rolled oats

A few pecans

Small amount low-fat natural yoghurt

Instructions

Preheat your oven to 200 °C (400 °F). On a baking tray, spread out the rolled oats and crush the pecans. Warm up the maple syrup, drizzle 2 teaspoons over the oats and nuts, and mix together. Smooth the ingredients out on your baking tray, and cook for 15 to 20 minutes until golden brown, stirring halfway through.

Peel the mango and orange and place in a blender. Add your small amount of low-fat natural yoghurt. Blend together, pour the mixture into a glass, and top with your homemade crunch.

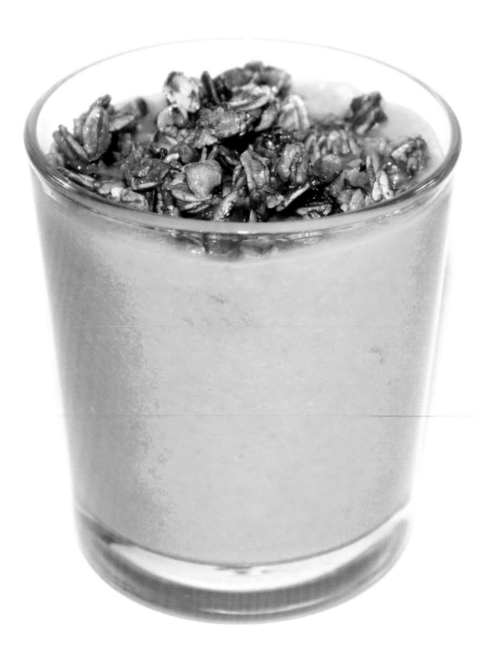

ANTI-AGING GRANOLA

A great way to feed your skin with the right vitamins and minerals every morning is by eating this homemade granola, which is very easy to make. You can make a big batch weekly and then store it in an airtight container. It will last for up to 10 days. You can also add in all sorts of extras, such as seeds, nuts or dried fruit, so experiment and get creative.

Ingredients

1 cup organic rolled oats

Handful of cranberries

Handful of raisins

Handful of pumpkin seeds

1 cup barley or rye flakes

Several crushed walnuts

3 tablespoons honey

Instructions

Preheat oven to 200 °C (400 °F). On a baking tray, spread out all the ingredients except the honey. Warm up the honey and pour evenly over the mixture. Then stir it and spread the mixture evenly over the baking tray. Place in the oven and bake for about 20 minutes or until golden brown, stirring halfway through.

I enjoy having this with some natural Greek yoghurt and sliced strawberries.

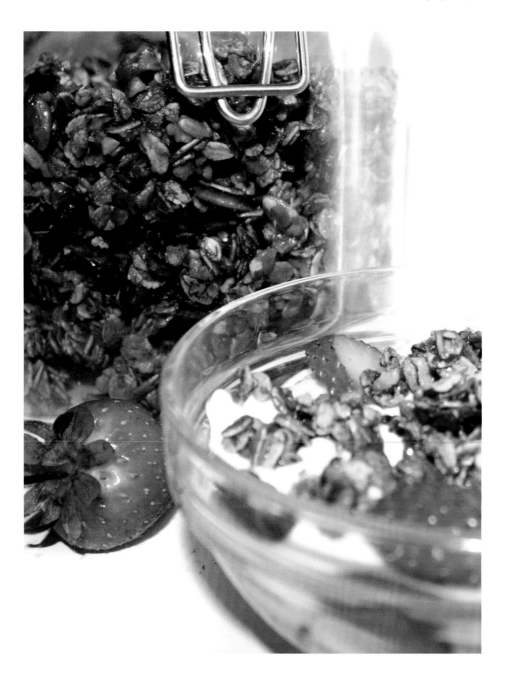

4

LOOK 10 YEARS YOUNGER GREEN SMOOTHIE

This smoothie just screams vitality and definitely makes you look 10 years younger, as it is rich in vitamins and minerals that care for your skin from inside out.

Ingredients

1/2 cucumber

2 celery sticks

Handful of spinach

1 carrot

1 pear

1 kiwi

1 apple

Instructions

Wash, peel, and chop all the ingredients. Put them into a blender and add a splash of water. If you like your smoothies super thick, only add a very small splash. Then blend and pour into a glass.

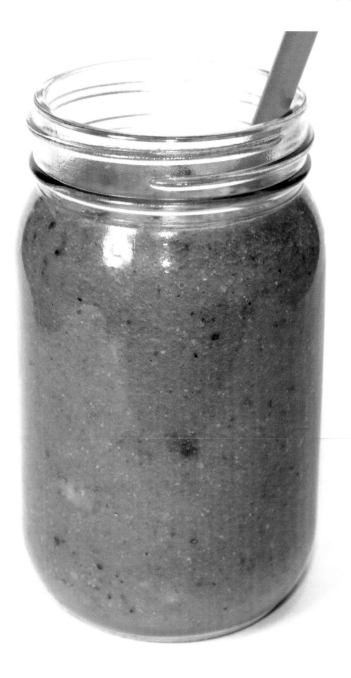

4

VELVET CHOCOLATE MOUSSE

The beauty of this anti-aging, creamy dessert is that it is perfect for any chocoholics who want to indulge guilt free. Also, every delicious mouthful is good for your skin, as the key ingredient, avocado (which you can't actually taste), is high in the good fats that help keep the skin plumped and glowing.

Ingredients

Avocado

Honey

2 tablespoons dark cocoa powder

Natural Greek yoghurt

Sprig of mint

1 raspberry

Instructions

Peel the avocado and remove the stone. Put it into a blender with some natural Greek yoghurt, dark cocoa powder, and honey. Blend until the mixture is a creamy consistency. Remove and pour into a bowl. Let it set for 10 minutes in the fridge. Top with your sprig of mint and a raspberry, and enjoy.

You can add a variety of toppings, and another one of my favourites to add is hazelnuts and pomegranates.

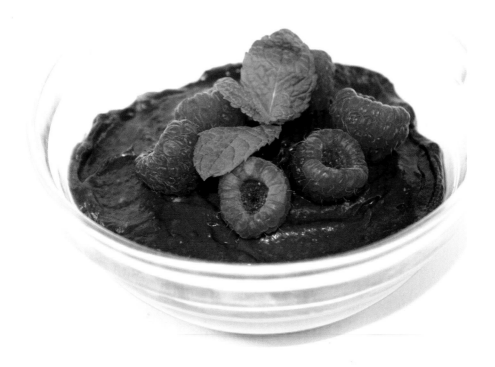

TIPS FOR MOTIVATION

Let's be honest, we are all going to have the odd day in which our motivation has dipped, and this can happen because we are tired, or maybe the weather is bad, or we lack energy. Whatever the reason, here are some top tips of mine on how you can instantly restore your motivation to 100 per cent.

Tip 1: Mind Makeover. Attitude is everything, so think of exercise and healthy eating as your daily dose of wellbeing. You know once you have had this you will feel great all day.

Tip 2: Put on Your Visualization Glasses. Take 5 minutes to sit down and visualise all the rewards you get from maintaining a healthy life, how great you will look in that new outfit, how you will have bundles of energy and even how glowing your skin, hair and nails will look. That is exactly how you can be with a healthy lifestyle.

Tip 3: Score a Goal. You have now accomplished one goal—following this book. So go on to set your own new goal. It could be as simple as in one month you aim to complete 12 walks and do your makeover motivation workout 10 times. You could have your goals as a tick list on your fridge.

Tip 4: Be Your Own Fitness DJ. Fact: music is the best motivator to get you in the mood for moving. It works. So every 21 days, update and refresh your workout playlist.

Tip 5: On the Dot. Find the best time of the day to work out and always try to stick to that. Some of us are naturally more energised in the morning, yet others feel more energy in the afternoon or evening. So find out your peak energy hour and make that your allocated workout time.

Tip 6: Become a Master Chef. Why not learn some new healthy recipes? The better your nutrition, then the more energy you will have, and the better you feel. So choose some of your favourite healthy natural ingredients and get cooking, and send me a picture of your healthy creation on Twitter or Instagram, @lucywyndhamread, #lucyhealthyfood.

CASE STUDIES

In the past 20 years, for me, the biggest buzz I get as a trainer has been when I receive emails, testimonials and even comments on my Instagram, YouTube and Twitter feed. I always want to deliver outstanding results and ensure that everyone who follows my workouts falls in love with leading a healthy lifestyle and gets the results they dream of.

Here are just some examples of what I have received. For more, please visit my website at www.lwrfitness.com/before-after. I will keep posting these motivational stories from around the world. Once you have finished this 21-day plan, please send me your story, hashtag: #lwrbeforeandafter.

4

CHARLIE PALLETT

Blogger

www.styledbycharlie.com

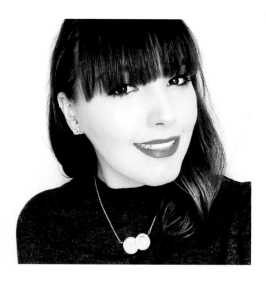

I've loved every minute of my training with Lucy. Her approach makes working out no longer a chore. It's fun and easy to adopt into any lifestyle. **I've lost 2 pounds each week**, and I'm so, so pleased!

Doing the workouts has become a new love for me! Doing short, sharp bursts of exercise has been such a wake-up call for me. Knowing I can now fit a workout into my busy day, easily targeting fitness and weight loss, has been my favourite change so far. I'm enjoying working out—I never thought I'd say that!

I've been documenting my health, fitness and weight-loss journey every Tuesday on my blog at www.styledbycharlie.com in a series called #TransformationTuesday, sharing my thoughts and tips for my readers. I want everyone to know that they can achieve a healthy and fit lifestyle by making just some minor lifestyle changes.

What has really stood out for me from Lucy's advice was that I've been eating more than I would when not on a diet and fitness plan, but I'm still losing weight. It's made me realise how important eating three times a day is and how essential it is to have a healthy and balanced lifestyle, and it's amazing how much effect it has on weight loss, health and fitness in a short period of time.

I feel great!

I've never felt more motivated to exercise and eat healthily; it's such a great programme, and I'm truly loving it!

4

GEMMA LOUISE HOMEBURY

Mum

I messaged Lucy in a desperate attempt for her expert advice, and out of the kindness of her heart, she took time to listen and find out what I wanted to achieve. Lucy designs workouts that work and eating plans that helped me get my diet right. The quick workouts I can do in the morning—I was blown away. Not only were the workouts intense, but I could fit one in before I had to do the school run for my other eldest daughter then again do another one once both my children were asleep. **I love Lucy's workouts**, and I can't thank her enough for helping me feel **comfortable in my skin again as well as confident**.

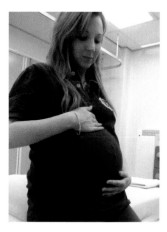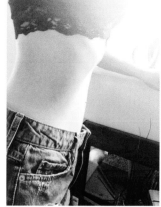

LIA VOONG

Working mum

Lucy's workouts are not only quick to do but also so simple. Being a mother of two and having three jobs, finding time to work out can be hard—until I came across Lucy's workouts. Now cannot thank her enough! Thank you, Lucy X.

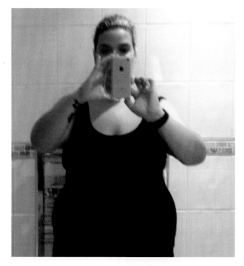

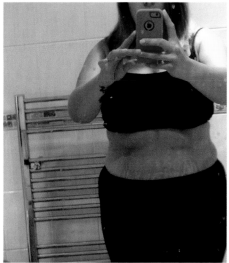

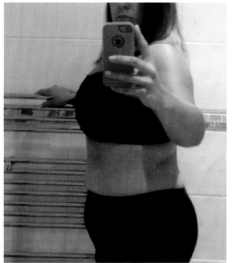

4

LIZZIE

Hi Lucy,

I saw your shout-out on Instagram, and thought I would write you a message.

I don't have any before or after pictures, but I wanted to let you know I am 31 and have a two-year-old daughter. A year and a half ago, I was diagnosed with thyroid cancer and have had ongoing treatments and surgeries, which included having my thyroid removed. All of this, coupled with having a very energetic little one, has left me feeling exhausted. Despite not being given the all-clear yet, my energy levels have greatly improved, and recently I've felt like I want to do some exercise. In the past I would go to classes or out running, but I just couldn't see myself fitting it around my daughter and my recovery.

As if by magic, I came across your YouTube channel, and I realised that I cannot only work out from home but fit in short, highly effective workouts that my rather battered body can cope with and easily recover from. Thanks to you, I see exercising in an entirely different light. Instead of thinking I need two spare hours to drag myself out to an exercise class, I can actually squeeze in a workout when my daughter naps or power walk to the park with her in the buggy. It feels fantastic to be taking such a positive step towards my recovery and feeling as though I have some more control over my health.

Thank you again for everything that you share. **You've really made a difference in my life**.

With all good wishes,

Lizzie

KAJAL

Working out used to be so daunting because I genuinely would not know where to start. Lucy's workouts may appear simple, but they really do pack a punch and send that heartbeat racing. I've noticed positive changes in not only my physical health, but my mental health, too. I cannot thank this lovely, motivational, relatable and inspiring lady enough for all she has done in the fitness world.

You, Lucy, are a star.

Thank you,

Kajal

AMY

Hi Lucy!

I want to thank you for all your help! I am a 22-year-old girl from New Zealand, and I've only been following your workouts for the last few weeks. In that time you have inspired me to get fit and healthy! I love your short simple workouts as I can get a workout in before I go to uni or work. In just the few weeks I've been watching, **I've lost 6 kilograms** and do not wanna stop! Your enthusiasm and short simple workouts have helped me fall in love with my new lifestyle!

Thank you so much, you are such a positive role model to all women out there!

Please never stop!

Amy

4

MEGAN

Hi Lucy!

I just wanted to give you an update. I've been sticking to eating good and exercising daily, and I can feel a difference! I love how short your workouts are. I actually started week 1 over again because I've been coming off a medicine, and I had bad insomnia, and I skipped my workouts last weekend all together, so I just started over. But I'm back on track now. I feel like my legs especially are getting more toned, which I love because that's my problem area. My tummy needs a lot of work, but I've noticed it's not as fluffy as it has been. I'm so thankful that you sent me your 21-day plan. I love it! I definitely feel the results, and I love how it gives me confidence. I know it'll take time to be where I want to be, but this has been the only workout that had ever made me feel it afterwards. It's very rewarding. I tried on a dress today that I couldn't fit into **6 months ago, and IT FITS**. I think I'm going to go shopping and buy something a size smaller for motivation so I can fit into it later. I'm so happy with how it's making me feel! Thank you so much!

Megan

LUCY'S INSPIRATION

The greatest man in my life is my wonderful dad, and he has taught me so much just from being the person he is.

Every single day, without fail, he walks between 40 minutes to an hour, and he is such a strong, focused and fit man. He is my world. My dad has always looked after his health and is a well-known folk singer with the most beautiful voice. He tours worldwide, so wherever he is in the world, if it is in America, Hong Kong or, his favourite, Australia, he will head out for his walk. http://www.martynwyndhamread.com

"Good health is real wealth." –Martyn Wyndham-Read

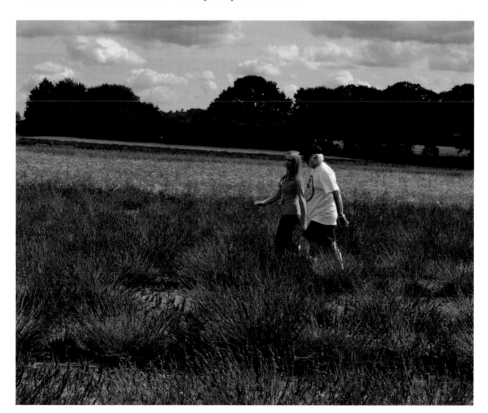

4

This picture was taken in 2014 when my dad climbed Snowdon! Also pictured are my wonderful cousin, Mark, and his beautiful wife.

A great example of the best thing in life—being fit.

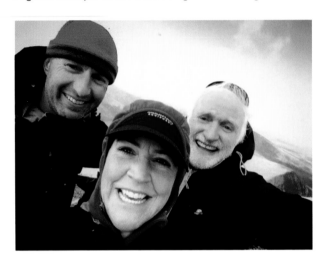

ACKNOWLEDGEMENTS

I first want to say a big thank-you to my wonderful mum, who has always been my mentor and keeps me driven and focused. She is such a beautiful woman, both inside and out. And thank you to my dad for giving me his drive. Thanks to my wonderful Uncle Keith, who has the great task of proofreading everything before I send to my publishers. (Each time I make fewer mistakes!) And thank you to the rest of my wonderful family: Jess, Johnny, Hatty, Tom, Mimi, Looby-Lou, Keith, Mandy, Ian, Joss, Cindy, Abigail, Mark, Alyna, and all the rest of my lovely family. You are all so special to me.

Then there are my dear friends, Michael, who has not only helped with the hectic filming schedules and long photo shoots but also been a true friend, and Rowan, who has always had faith in me, told me my dreams would come true and has supported me in many ways. And, finally, Tony Stevens, for all the great indoor fitness pictures.

In life the most important things are FAMILY, FRIENDS, FITNESS and FOOD.

Finally, a special acknowledgement to my fiancé who was sadly taken from me but has always been my shining star and who I believe has been my guardian angel in life. Every book I do, I dedicate to him.

4

GET IN TOUCH

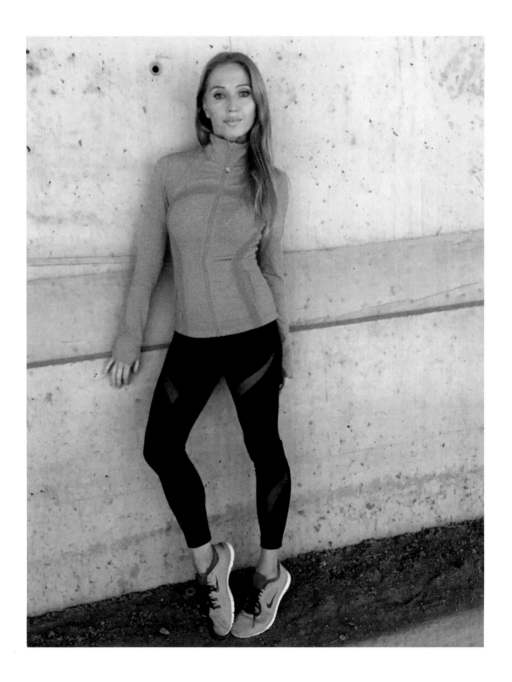

Let me know how you get on with this 21-day plan of mine and send me your before and after pictures.

Twitter		Tweet me @lucywyndhamread
Pinterest		Pin me a picture @LWR Fitness
Facebook		Like me and share your pics with me @LWR Fitness
Instagram		Follow me @lucywyndhamread

For weekly workouts, motivation and so much more, head to my YouTube Channel at

LWRFitness: YOUTUBE.COM/LWRFitnessChannel

CREDITS

Cover, jacket design, layout and typesetting:		Sannah Inderelst
Graphic:	jacket:	© Thinkstock/iStock/AppleEyesStudio
	p. 26, 27, 40:	© Thinkstock/iStock
	p. 136:	© Thinkstock/iStock

Photos:

Cover photo:	Tony Stevens
Indoor exercises:	Tony Stevens
Food, lifestyle, and outdoor photos:	Michael Lloyd at MensFitKitchen.com and Lucy Wyndham-Read
Editing:	Elizabeth Evans